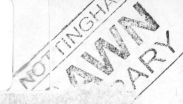
Loss, bereavement and grief

A guide to effective caring

Bob Spall and Stephen Callis

Stanley Thornes (Publishers) Ltd

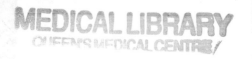
First published 1997 by:
Stanley Thornes (Publishers) Ltd
Ellenborough House
Wellington Street
CHELTENHAM
GL50 1YW
United Kingdom

97 98 99 00 01 / 10 9 8 7 6 5 4 3 2 1

A catalogue record for this book is available from the British Library
ISBN 0–7487–3322–1

Typset by Florencetype Ltd, Stoodleigh, Devon
Printed and bound in Great Britain by
TJ International, Padstow, Cornwall

To Hilary, Jonathan, Matthew and Rebecca
To Val, Clare, Katherine and Gillian

Contents

Preface

The initial ideas for this book arose out of a series of workshops on loss, death and bereavement conducted by the authors in the early 1990s. These were for a wide range of helping professionals and it became apparent that there was a need for a book which focused on what it meant to be an effective helper in practice. Such a book would need to make links between theory, personal loss issues and professional practice.

Bob Spall changed his job in 1993 and this was an impetus to begin shaping up the original ideas for the book. Work following this transition proved to be both a valuable learning experience and relevant to the content of the book. It has included being on working parties and involvement in training in relation to improving palliative care within the North Staffordshire Combined Healthcare NHS Trust. In addition, Bob Spall has learned much from being associated with the Bereavement Care organization in Hanley, Stoke-on-Trent over the last 4 years.

Stephen Callis has recently completed an MA in counselling studies at Keele University. This has also been a useful learning experience which has aided the writing of the book. There has been the added stimulation of academic life, together with the opportunity of talking over issues with fellow students (several of whom worked in health-care settings) and with staff.

This book is intended for nurses, doctors, social workers and other professional helpers who work with people experiencing loss. It is the result of a meeting of minds with different perspectives and experiences. Bob Spall has been a practising clinical psychologist for 19 years and Stephen Callis has been a hospital chaplain and a practising counsellor for over 20 years.

It will be noted that the terms 'patient' and 'client' are used interchangeably, depending on the context. Also, in Chapter 1, where the loss experiences of several different people are described, first names (which are fictitious) are used in order to make discussing comparisons between them easier. In subsequent chapters, people are referred to by their job or kind of work.

In using the book, readers are recommended to make links between theory, the experience of other professionals and their own practice, and also to consider connections between personal and professional issues. This process is aided in two ways.

- There are questions at the end of some chapters which aim to trigger thinking about these issues.
- In some chapters, questions to consider are raised within the body of the text.

Some of these questions may be difficult to address and it is recommended that thoughts about them be shared with a colleague. This will help to share any stress involved and also to learn from each other.

In order to cover all the areas that are important in relation to the provision of effective care, it is suggested that the book be read through rather than 'dipped into'. Being able to work effectively with people facing loss is an enormous challenge, as it can raise difficult personal and professional issues. It is hoped that this book will assist the reader in meeting that challenge.

KEY WORDS

Throughout the process of writing this book the authors have borne in mind the important question: in working with loss, what is required to be an effective helping professional? Certain key words have helped us to stay focused on this question and express in essence what the book is about:

- **appreciation** that change and loss includes minor loss and is part of everyday life; also that the world of work is changing and stressful, making a sense of personal value very important; in addition, appreciating how expectations associated with 'being professional' can increase stress;
- **understanding** the normal emotional processes that can occur in loss, bereavement and dying so that we might work with them and avoid pitfalls such as taking reactions personally; also, understanding of the spiritual dimension as well as the specifically religious and cultural;
- **personal insights** into how both experienced and feared loss can affect work – this also includes considering one's own mortality; such personal insights inevitably involve making links between personal and professional issues;
- **skills** such as those involved in communication and basic counselling are required to break bad news, work with collusion or enable

unfinished business; such skills are also important in recognising the need to refer on;

- **support** for ourselves so that we can maintain the emotional energy needed to work with people facing loss – this includes formal and informal support – and also supporting oneself, by maintaining a sense of balance and some boundaries between working and non-working lives.

It will be recognized from this range of issues that we are concerned with addressing the interaction between professional and personal spheres and how this can affect working with loss. We feel that it is important to stress that this book is grounded in reality. It draws on information collected in individual interviews, in which the following groups have been represented: medicine (physician, surgeon and psychiatrist), nursing (general and psychiatric), social work, clinical psychology, counselling, chaplaincy, teaching, hospital support workers, and voluntary sector workers. We have also made use of insights and data gained from numerous workshops with helping professionals and from the use of some questionnaires.

Acknowledgements

There are many people who have enlightened us during the course of writing this book. We are very grateful to those from various professions who agreed to be interviewed and were very open about their professional and personal experiences of loss. In order to retain confidentiality, these people cannot be named. However, we hope they will notice that many of their thoughts and experiences have been incorporated into the book.

We are also indebted to the many professionals who have attended our workshops over the past few years. They have taught us a great deal from their wealth of experience and have helped us to develop our ideas. Another important group who have helped to teach us about the nature of loss are the clients and their relatives whom we have seen over the years in our different professional contexts.

Numerous people have engaged in informal discussion of ideas with us. We would particularly like to thank Alison Rawle, clinical nurse specialist, Rev. Godfrey Stone, hospital chaplain, Sue Booth, palliative care nurse and Pat Mood and Margaret Foulkes, both hospice social workers. On a broader level we are grateful to Alison Norman, executive director – nursing/clinical director of primary care, who has enabled us to learn from the palliative care initiatives of the North Staffs Combined Healthcare NHS Trust over the last three to four years. Also, to senior nursing/managerial staff in the East Cheshire NHS Trust who originally involved us in their terminal care work in the early 1990s.

Members of the Bereavement Care Research Forum (Hanley, Stoke-on-Trent) have also engaged in helpful discussion with us. In particular we would like to thank Irene Frost who has helped to stimulate our ideas on feared loss and Grace Jordan who has assisted us in understanding some loss issues for teachers, via a questionnaire survey. We are grateful to those teachers who responded to the questionnaire.

Various library staff have been helpful to us, particularly in the early stages of researching material for the book. We would like to thank librarians at the following libraries: North Staffordshire Medical Institute, Department of Nursing and Midwifery at the University of Keele and the Halley Stewart library at St Christopher's Hospice, Sydenham, London.

We would like to acknowledge the help of Rosemary Morris, Associate Publisher, who encouraged us to pursue our ideas about the book when we first approached Chapman & Hall in 1994. Also, the help of Neal Marriott, List Development Manager, who ensured a smooth transition when Chapman & Hall's health sciences list was transferred to Stanley Thornes.

Finally, we have written this book while at the same time maintaining busy working lives. It would not have been possible without the support and tolerance of our wives and children. We are grateful to them for helping to turn our idea for the book into a reality.

Bob Spall
Stephen Callis

Looking at change in our lives

1

It's a risk to attempt new beginnings ... Yet the greater risk is for you to risk nothing. For there will be no further possibilities of learning and changing, of travelling upon the journey of life.

Grollman, 1987

Death is not the only loss that calls for grieving ... It is equally important to mourn the death of a relationship when a divorce occurs, the loss of familiar surroundings when relocating to another city, the loss of a job ...

Deits, 1992

What we have found remarkable is how apparently ordinary people achieve extraordinary wisdom through their struggle with circumstances that are initially aversive in the extreme.

Tedeschi and Calhoun, 1995

We all experience periods of change and transition in our lives, for example starting or changing school, starting a job, leaving home and developing a close relationship. Often the stress of change is associated with negative or unpleasant events such as losing a job. However, positive or pleasant events can also require considerable adjustment, for example getting married, the birth of a child or promotion at work. This is reflected in the early work of Holmes and Rahe (1967) on life events, referred to later in this chapter. There can be gains as well as losses in any change and many authors have alluded to this. Tedeschi and Calhoun (1995) suggest that living through life traumas can result, for example, in increased self-reliance and personal strength, positive changes in relationships with others and an increased appreciation of life. Ward (1993) points to positive gain for some parents of disabled children: 'They see their "special" child as having brought out from within themselves an understanding, joy and compassionate love that they would not otherwise have experienced.'

A more general example of gain as well as loss is when grown up children leave home. There is loss for the parents (sometimes referred to as 'the empty nest') but on the other hand there can be a new sense of freedom for parents who may have been putting their children's needs first for over 20 years.

The Chinese have two symbols for crisis, one indicating danger and the other opportunity. The danger is that someone will be unable to cope and be psychologically damaged by the experience. The opportunity is for personal growth, which can be achieved if loss is successfully worked through and advantage is taken of potential gains. People who have experienced major loss may become more compassionate and understanding. Often people with serious, life-threatening illness talk of changed priorities; for example, material things become unimportant while relationships become more significant. An elderly patient seen by one of the authors had been married for over 50 years and was trying to come to terms with her husband's sudden, severe stroke, which resulted in long-term hospitalization. They had done most things together and she described a 'gain' in the process of trying to build a more independent life. She talked in terms of having to think 'I' instead of 'We' and was learning to rely more on her personal resources.

In this chapter we will be considering how change, minor as well as major, can affect people and illustrating a common thread of reactions. Difficulties that can arise in adjusting to transitions will also be discussed. The reader may find it helpful to contemplate general changes in his/her own life in relation to the content of this chapter.

REACTIONS TO 'MINOR' LOSS

Loss and the consequent emotional reactions are frequently associated with something major such as a bereavement. What happens when something less traumatic occurs? Do people just shrug it off? Jane, an occupational therapist, was working on a project on her computer and was going through a process to make more room on the disc before she could save her work. She pressed a particular button and immediately became aware that she might have lost her work (2–3 hours' worth). She thought, 'I haven't lost that, have I?' and begun to have palpitations and a sense of fear that the work had gone. This had happened before and she had a feeling of *déjà vu*. She brought the file up, pressed the down cursor and began to experience shock and disbelief, thinking, 'Its got to be there!'

As Jane started to resign herself to the fact that her work was not there she swore at the computer and tried to blame her partner for what had happened ('If only we had a better computer!'). She didn't want to believe it was her fault. She was angry that the work had gone; there was a time pressure to finish the work so time was precious and she had wasted it. There was then a feeling of hope: 'Maybe it's in limbo and I can retrieve it?' Although it was 12.20 am she thought perhaps she could telephone a friend who would know what to do. She didn't care if she disturbed him; it was worth risking it as the computer couldn't be left on all night. Next there was a feeling of catastrophe that the work had actually gone. As the realization that she had lost the work began to sink in, Jane thought, 'I don't deserve this, I'm a good person. Why has this happened to me?'

After this Jane tried to get things in perspective: 'It's not the end of the world, nobody has died. The work has not gone for ever as I was working from notes. It'll take another 2–3 hours; the only thing I've lost is the time.' However, she still felt very irritated by what had happened. The reactions she described lasted for about 45 minutes.

The feeling of irritation/anger continued the next day and she was dreading having to put the work back on the computer, partly because she was bored with it and didn't want to have to do it again. However, she did the work again that day and when she got to the point where she had lost all the work the previous night there was a sense of relief. It had been retrieved, the loss had been put right and she could move on from here.

The reader may be thinking that Jane had really got things out of proportion here and made a mountain out of a molehill. However, the emotional reactions she describes, shock, disbelief, 'why me?', anxiety, anger, hope, a feeling that the loss has been resolved and being able to move on, are all normal reactions to loss described, for example, by Parkes (1996) and Marris (1986).

Let us take another non-major loss to illustrate how common and normal such emotional reactions are. This example is used in the Open University pack on death and dying (Open University, 1992). Bram, a university tutor, had his wallet stolen and his first reaction was disbelief: 'Perhaps it is in my back pocket or I've put it down somewhere.' He then felt shock and talked of two particular things in the wallet that were important to him: a small picture of his father (the only copy of that particular photograph) and a page of a letter written to him by a friend. Following this he felt angry and cross. Apart from losing the valuable items and £40, it was so inconvenient. He then asked, 'Why me? There are plenty of other people around,' and felt frustrated as he had things to do. Feelings of this kind lasted to the end of the day. Subsequently, he felt dejected and wished it hadn't happened. Thoughts then arose about who was to blame: was it the security system or perhaps he should blame himself for being absent-minded. He might never get the valuable mementos back. Bram's reactions of disbelief, shock, anger, 'why me?', frustration, dejection and looking for someone to blame are very similar to Jane's reactions to losing her work on the computer.

A GENERAL MODEL OF CHANGE

Moving on to consider transition and change in general, Hopson (1981) has presented a model of how mood or self-esteem changes with time during a transition (Figure 1.1).

These changes are likely to occur when something happens (or doesn't happen, such as a couple failing to conceive a planned baby) that leads to a change in assumptions about ourselves and the world. The model is described below.

- **Immobilization**. This can be equated with shock or a sense of being overwhelmed. If you discovered that your car had been stolen, your first reaction might be 'It can't have gone' or 'I must have parked it somewhere else'. Similarly, if you inherited a great deal of money that you had not been expecting you might think 'This can't be happening to me. There must be some mistake'.
- **Reaction**
  Elation or despair. After the sense of shock, mood can change according to the type of transition that has been experienced. For something pleasant or desired this could range from mild positive feelings up to elation. If the event was unpleasant or undesired, mood could range from being a little disappointed to very despondent or depressed.

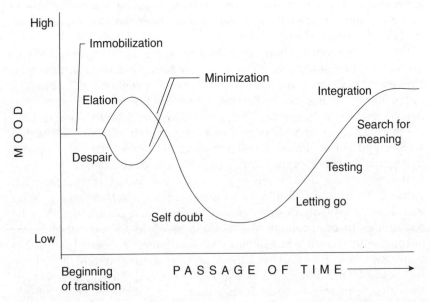

Figure 1.1 Cycle of reactions and feelings accompanying transition (reproduced from Sugarman, 1986, with permission; adapted from Hopson, 1981).

Minimization. For a positive event such as a promotion at work the initial feelings of elation may be followed by thoughts such as 'Will I be able to cope?' or 'How will the extra pressure affect my life outside of work?' A negative event such as a period of a few weeks' illness may be accompanied by thoughts like 'I can do some reading that I normally never have time to do' or 'I can have some peace and quiet for a change'. Thus when the other side of a positive transition becomes apparent the initial feelings of elation will probably be dampened down. With a negative change the effect of the event may be played down: it may be seen as less grim than it was initially.

- **Self-doubt**. As the reality of how one's world is different becomes apparent a period of self-doubt ensues. For some people this may be experienced as depression. Other associated feelings might include anger and anxiety. Energy levels may also vary; for instance the person may fluctuate between feeling apathetic and angry.

- **Letting go**. Accepting the reality of change is a significant point in a transition and probably the most difficult. It involves beginning to let go of attachments to the past and facing the future. This mourning for the loss of the past may be accompanied by feelings of upset and anger at the injustice of it all. It is from this point on that the possibility of personal growth emerges, learning from negative events in our lives so that we become more mature individuals.

- **Testing**. This is a period of considering possibilities for the future. Some things may be tried and then dropped. New skills and new behaviours may be required during this experimental period as attachments to the new world begin to be formed. There may be mood changes, e.g. when plans don't work out, but on the whole mood or self-esteem will be increasing.

- **Search for meaning**. During this phase people are actively trying to make sense of the experience and to learn from it. They may be asking questions such as 'What does all this mean for me and my future?'

- **Integration**. When people feel at ease in their new world and are comfortable with the new demands and behaviours required of them, the phase of integration has been achieved.

Clearly this is a general model and it cannot be expected that everyone experiencing a transition will pass smoothly through these phases. People may progress to one stage and then revert to an earlier phase. For some transitions people may get stuck and never progress beyond the early stages.

ADJUSTMENT TO CHANGE: THE EXAMPLE OF REDUNDANCY

In relation to this model, consider the example of Alan (in his early 50s), who was an engineer for a large organization and had worked there for many years. His wife was very worried about the possibility of his being made redundant. Alan's work base was due to close, and his job ceased to exist. He was made redundant quickly and unexpectedly, being given only 2 days notice. He finished work on a Friday and on the following Monday he started attending an out-placement agency with staff and other resources to help him find another job.

Alan was allocated a counsellor at the agency, whom he only wanted to see very briefly, and he then worked on his own. It was common for people to attend the agency for 2–3 hours at a time. However, Alan attended all day, every day and seemed to be regarding himself as part of the counselling team. He was not really doing a lot while he was there. After about 4 weeks he appeared morose and remote and when his counsellor talked to him, it transpired that he had not told his family that he had been made redundant. He had pretended that he was going to work as usual, leaving and returning at his normal time. Apart from being worried about his job situation, his wife was still experiencing psychological difficulties in relation to the death of one of their children 2 years previously. Alan's relationship with his wife was strained and he was afraid of telling her about his redundancy in case she 'broke down' and/or left him.

Alan was immobilized by the shock of being made redundant with only 2 days notice and was unable to make proper use of the outplacement agency during the first few weeks. He minimized the event by pretending that it hadn't happened; he was denying the reality of the situation. His later moroseness and remoteness could be linked with the depression of self-doubt.

After talking to the counsellor Alan told his wife and began to come into the agency less over the next few months. He was beginning to let go of his old situation and exploring new job possibilities. After a few months he secured another job that made use of his skills. As he settled into his new job he reached the stage of integration. Some of the gains in this situation were that Alan obtained a new and interesting job, which had prospects, and of course he obtained a good redundancy package.

Another example will help to illustrate the model further. Hazel was a book-keeper for a medium-sized company and the business was not going too well. Somebody new (who happened to be a personal friend of the boss) was taken on and Hazel trained her. Then one morning Hazel went into work and was told that her services were no longer required as the company couldn't afford to employ her any more. Within half an hour she was on her way home again.

For 2 days she was in a state of shock and disbelief. She then became very irritated that this woman friend of the boss (who was cheaper to employ) was being kept on and was livid that she couldn't do anything about what had happened. During this time if her young son committed some misdemeanour, she would over-react and become very angry. She felt like putting a brick through a window of her ex-employers and also wanted to pick up the telephone and shout at them. Two brothers-in-law worked for the same company and neither of them said anything to her; she was left with a feeling of being let down.

Hazel quickly applied for other jobs and within weeks she was working in a new job. What helped her to let go of the old job was the fact that her new job was much more interesting. She had taken the whole event personally and hadn't considered the financial situation of the previous company. Thus she was beginning to make sense of what had happened. Apart from the gain of a more interesting job, there were other gains subsequent to Hazel's transition. Later on her husband was made redundant and was without a job for 6–7 months and she was able to support him through this experience. Also, in her later work in redundancy counselling she could relate to her clients' feelings of anger, rejection, having no control and uncertainty.

A TASK MODEL

Worden (1991) describes the process of adjusting to bereavement in terms of tasks of mourning and this will be considered in Chapter 7. However, to illustrate that this model can be applied to losses other than bereavement, we will discuss it now in relation to the kind of job losses described above.

Task one is to accept the reality of the loss. For Alan it took over a month before he could begin to face the reality of losing his job. By comparison Hazel appears to have begun facing her loss within a few days.

Task two is to work through the pain of grief. Alan seemed to be morose and remote and Hazel experienced extreme irritation and anger: she felt things were out of her control and that she had been let down. Losing a job may entail, for example, experiencing the pain of rejection, loss of identity or reduction in self-esteem, reduction in interpersonal contacts and loss of a sense of belonging (see, for example, Warr, 1987a). People who have been made redundant may avoid thinking about their loss by engaging in comfort spending or frenetic activity involving, for example, DIY, sport and travel.

Task three in this work-related context is to adjust to an environment in which the job is missing. This may entail learning new skills and looking to possibilities for work in the future in an attempt to regain some control of life.

Task four is to put the job loss in perspective and be able to move on with life. This may be achieved when a new job is obtained (especially if, as in the above cases, the new job is in some ways better than the old one) or when there is an increased value attached to other aspects of life, e.g. voluntary work, family life, education or hobbies.

REFLECTING ON A TRANSITION CHART: THE EXAMPLE OF A PSYCHIATRIC NURSE

Another way of looking at change in our lives is to consider our own life line. This has been described, for example, by Machin (1990) and Lendrum and Syme (1992). Essentially it involves marking off significant transitions such as job changes and family births and deaths on a time line ranging from birth to one's current age.

We have modified this approach by including a rating of the degree of adjustment required or the degree of distress caused by each transition. Elaine is a trained psychiatric nurse and a chart showing some of her transitions is shown in Figure 1.2. As indicated, the transitions marked with an asterisk all occurred within the space of 18 months, so the chart is not to scale.

A glance at Figure 1.2 will indicate that Elaine has experienced more life events than many 42-year-olds. A lot of people of this age may, for example, still not have experienced the death of a close relative.

By discussing Elaine's reactions to some of her life transitions we will indicate the similarities with the reactions to more minor losses described earlier in this chapter. Also, Elaine's experiences of multiple

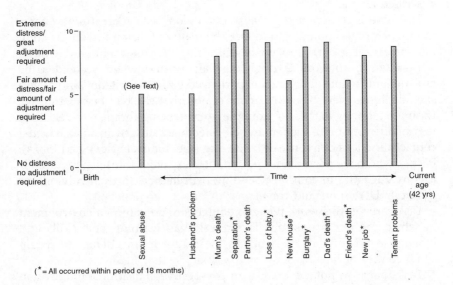

Figure 1.2 Elaine's life transitions chart – degree of distress or adjustment associated with each transition.

life transitions and the problems these have caused in relation to adjustment to change will be discussed in relation to the models of Hopson
(1981) and Worden (1991). In addition, we will mention some of her
coping strategies.

One difficulty about estimating with hindsight the degree of distress
caused by, or adjustment required after, a transition is that how we
thought about it at the time may be very different to how we think
about it now. This was the case with Elaine's recollection of being sexu-
ally abused as a teenager. Initially she had not put this on the chart. 'I
don't know why I haven't put it on – perhaps because I don't want to
talk about it.' When talking about going through the experience she said,
'At the time I just seemed to go along with it . . . I wasn't particularly
frightened.' Her rating of the experience was 5 or 6 on the scale, which
indicates a fair amount of distress/required adjustment. However, she
finds it traumatic to think about it now and feels extremely angry about
what happened. 'I feel absolutely intense hatred towards him: I could
kill him.' On the 10-point scale she gives a rating of 12 (off the scale) to
indicate the severe difficulties this transition is still causing her. (In
looking at any transition chart or life line, this kind of discrepancy
indicates unfinished business.)

Elaine's husband was accused of (and admitted to) indecent as-
sault and she couldn't believe it. When the police came to the door
she couldn't understand what was going on. The next day she just
wandered around the shops with her children. 'I went into total shock,
I was numb, I really felt numb.' She had flu and took to her bed for
a week. She never forgave him and couldn't see him in the same
light again.

She separated from her husband and, with a new partner, Donald,
was in the process of buying a house together when he committed
suicide. This was very traumatic and for a while she felt suicidal. 'It was
just the complete shock of it all, shock horror of it. I couldn't believe
that this bloke, who'd been telling me that we were going to be married
and have a baby and start a new life together, had gone and done this.'
Her disbelief was further echoed in her statement: 'This was a bloke of
35, he'd got everything to live for.' Her feelings of anger towards Donald
are exacerbated by her belief that he contributed to the death of her
father. 'I feel so much anger towards Donald, it's unbelievable. As time
goes on I'm getting more and more angry towards him.' She expressed
her difficulty in coping with the suicide: 'I really don't think I ever will
come to terms with it, I don't think I can.'

The picture becomes more complicated in that Elaine feels she also
contributed to her father's death. After Donald's death, when she was
feeling suicidal, she reported putting her dad through hell. She feels
very, very guilty about this.

A COMMON THREAD OF REACTIONS TO LOSS

Let us stop to reflect for a while on some of Elaine's reactions and feelings. Just as in the earlier examples of reactions to minor loss, she has experienced shock and anger but the difference seems to be a question of degree. She uses terms like 'total shock', 'really felt numb', 'I feel so much anger, it's unbelievable' and 'intense hatred'. (N.B. In relation to the anger, she also reports, 'I think, "God, why have I been left in this mess?" ' This 'Why me?' is similar to the earlier examples of reactions to minor loss.) In the previously discussed examples of job loss and minor loss, guilt was not highlighted, although it may have been around in relation to taking anger out on family members. By comparison Elaine talks in terms of feeling 'very, very guilty'.

EXTENT OF ADJUSTMENT: GETTING STUCK

When asked whether she had learnt anything about herself as a result of her experiences, Elaine's response was: 'I'm not the person I was: I'm not me any more.' She used to look at life differently; she used to joke and laugh. Now she gets very low, very irritable and, as mentioned above, is very, very angry. In relation to the Hopson model she appears to be stuck at the stage of the emotional reactions associated with self-doubt. She is unable to disentangle herself from the past, so is unable to begin letting go.

In terms of Worden's model, she has not properly worked through the pain of grief (task 2); in particular, there is a lot of unexpressed and unresolved anger. Part of the problem is the multiplicity of transitions Elaine has experienced; often another has come upon her before she has had a chance to resolve the previous one. She has not been able to work through tasks 3 and 4, i.e. to adjust to her new environment or move on with life. However, there have been some gains from her experiences – for example being able to relate better to bereaved people or those who have been burgled. The reader will recall that Hazel also gained from her experience of being made redundant in relation to being able to support others in a similar situation. This area of learning and gaining from personal loss, already referred to at the beginning of this chapter, will be expanded upon in Chapter 4.

LIFE EVENTS: THE CAUSES OF DYSFUNCTIONAL STRESS?

The reader may well be familiar with life events scales, as they are often quoted in relation to transition and change. Table 1.1 shows some of Elaine's transitions, all of which occurred within a period of about 1 year.

Table 1.1   A sample of Elaine's life events, all of which occurred within 1 year, and scores that would be allocated on Holmes and Rahe's social readjustment rating scale (Holmes and Rahe, 1967)

Life event/transition	Allocated score
Death of partner	100
Death of relative	63
Personal illness	53
Illness of relative	44
Pregnancy	40
Death of friend	37
Change of job	36
Change in standard of living	25
Change in job routine	20
Moving house	20
Change in sleeping habits	16
Change in frequency of family contacts	15
Total score	469

The scores that would be allocated to these events on the Holmes and Rahe (1967) social readjustment rating scale are also shown. The total score is 469. According to Holmes and Rahe, a score of over 300 in any one year puts a person at high risk of developing serious illness. Although Elaine did not develop a physical illness, she did become very depressed.

A problem with such scales is that they take no account of an individual's perspective on events. For example, Elaine found it very difficult to come to terms with changes in the frequency of family contacts. As she had joint custody of her children, they were only with her for half the week. 'Eighteen years with your children is a long time. I can't get used to them not being around every day.' She also talked of a great sense of loss in relation to her partner's family, as since his death she did not really feel part of it any more.

We do not find the disease perspective on life events and transitions particularly helpful. The assumption underlying the Holmes and Rahe scale is that life events are pathological and the causes of dysfunctional stress, which leads on to health problems. The approach would suggest that one should either try to avoid the occurrence of too many life events or deal with the stress caused. This then allows normal development. By comparison, the developmental perspective on transitions, which we discussed earlier in this chapter (e.g. Hopson, 1981) suggests a potential for personal growth as well as possible negative outcomes.

COPING STRATEGIES

One of the coping strategies referred to by Hopson (1981) is to know your anchor points. This involves holding on to something stable when all around is changing. Even though changing jobs was one of her later transitions, Elaine appeared to regard work as her anchor point. She went back to work 2 weeks after Donald's death. 'I used to get to the door of the ward and I used to say, "Right, this is your job now." ' She also commented, 'I've got no structure to my life any more. The only thing that I can hold on to is work; it's the only thing that is stable, really.'

Elaine reported that her friends have helped her most. 'I just bend their ear all the time; they're probably sick of me.' Also, after Donald's death she always had somebody around her (family or friends). Hence, her coping strategies included what Carver *et al.* (1989) refer to as seeking emotional social support (getting sympathy or emotional support from someone) and seeking instrumental social support (seeking assistance, information or advice about what to do). She did attend counselling sessions for a while and feels it may have helped her a little but, as mentioned above, feels pessimistic that she will ever be able to come to terms with all that has happened. She does accept, however, that if she could get rid of some of her anger it might help. She has outbursts when she is horrible and she never used to be like that.

COPING AND ASSOCIATION WITH OTHER LOSSES

Space does not permit us to describe all Elaine's experiences. However, some of her transitions do illustrate how a loss can be made more difficult to cope with by its association with other losses. For example, when she was burgled, 'they took my mum's Doulton figures, which meant a lot to me'. In relation to problems with the tenants in her parents' house (including damage to the house and going to court) she reported, 'I feel as if they've marred my mum and dad's memory.' When her 29-year-old friend with a young son died of cancer, she found it difficult to grieve for her because of connections she made with unresolved anger about Donald's death. 'I was so angry. Donald had gone and killed himself and somebody like her, who'd got everything to live for, had been mutilated by this disease. And I thought, "How dare he go and kill himself!" '

In this chapter we have illustrated how reactions and feelings associated with a wide range of changes are similar in nature. We have also looked at models that help to explain the work that needs to be done in adjusting to change, and considered the potential for gains and personal growth. Hopefully the reader will have made connections with his or her own experience and will perhaps have drawn up a transition chart. Other aspects of loss including its relationship to the concept of attachment will be explored in Chapter 7.

Working in a sea of change

2

How do you get senior colleagues to notice you are suffering from acute burnout? Do you send a memo or collapse in tears? . . . I want to be bright and helpful but instead I am prickly and defensive. I feel dispensable, disposable and despondent.

Letter in Community Care, June, 1984

When I see my boss coming over to talk to me, or even if he calls me on the phone, then I know it will be to point out some shortcomings or fault . . . The end result can be very very destructive and disheartening. I would dearly love to hear my boss say 'you really did a great job today'. But if I did I think I would drop through the floor.'

Clinical teacher quoted in Hingley and Cooper, 1986

One day my young patient with AIDS greeted me at the door with ". . . I really need the ray of sunshine and good cheer you always impart when you come to see me . . ." And with that he gave me a big hug. It really made my day, and I felt good about everything all day long – good and bad.

Caregiver quoted in Larson, 1993

Most professionals within the helping professions work in organizations, whose climate and culture may be subject to enormous changes. These can be affected by government policy, by a change in senior management and by general changes in the world of work. It is unlikely, for example, that many people now regard their work as secure, i.e. as 'a job for life.' Uncertainty about change and the accompanying feelings of insecurity can lead to high levels of stress. Professional helpers do not exist in a vacuum and have to work in this changing, uncertain environment.

This chapter considers some of the factors that will enable the reader to survive and work effectively in this environment. The areas we will consider are:

- understanding organizational change and stress;
- reducing the chances of becoming burnt out;
- coping generally with the stress of change;
- maintaining a sense of self-worth and value.

The important area of support for ourselves will be touched on but will be covered in more detail in Chapter 16. Connections will also be made with Chapter 3, on being professional. Working with people experiencing loss can be very difficult at times and if we are not coping with the other stresses around us it is unlikely that we will have any spare 'emotional energy' to work effectively with the dying, the bereaved and those experiencing other forms of loss.

UNDERSTANDING ORGANIZATIONAL CHANGE AND STRESS

Before considering sources of stress, we will consider some of the potential gains or benefits from work. Cook and Wall (1980), drawing on the work of Maslow, view work as meeting four areas of need:

- **social**, e.g. friendly contact with other people;
- **self-esteem**, e.g. prestige of job or recognition received for achievements;
- **autonomy**, e.g. making decisions about how you do the work;
- **self-actualization**, e.g. being able to extend your abilities further.

Another way of looking at the benefits of work is to consider what would be missing if one didn't have a job. Warr (1987b) considers several likely psychological effects, including loss of variety, loss of traction or structure and more insecurity (as well as not fulfilling the needs described by Cook and Wall above, e.g. decreased scope for decisions and less skill development). Other potential gains from work might include peer group respect, the opportunity to be creative and consciousness of bringing benefit to others.

It is worth stopping for a moment to reflect that stress is not just caused by external events but can also be influenced by how we perceive/appraise situations. This is the interactional view of stress described, for example, by Lazarus and Folman (1984). In later sections of this chapter we will also consider how problems with interpersonal skills and personality factors can contribute to stress. However, to return to the perspective of considering potential gains from work, stress is very likely to be experienced when achievement of some of the benefits of work is threatened.

We will now consider some of the factors in organizations that can work against the achievement of the benefits described above.

UNCERTAINTY ABOUT ONE'S ROLE

If we are not clear about the scope of our responsibility or about other people's expectations of how we should perform our job, this is likely to lead to feelings of insecurity. If we are not clear about how our work is evaluated, how can we know if we have done a good job? This is referred to as **role ambiguity**. The reader might like to reflect on some of these issues, for example:

- Am I clear about my role – what it involves and what it does not involve?
- Am I clear about the scope of my responsibilities?
- Do I know how my performance of my job will be evaluated?

The last example should be addressed in a proper individual performance review system. However, such reviews may not always be carried out in a balanced and professional manner. Hingley and Cooper (1986) quote a nursing sister:

> I absolutely dread reviews. In my experience it always degenerates into something which feels like the third degree ... It should provide the safety and support in which we can identify our weaknesses and build upon our strengths. Often it just seems to be a check-list of faults and shortcomings. It feels a bit like going through an MOT test. The fear of 'failure' is always there, often not very far beneath the surface.

Lack of clarity or misconceptions about role can result in lack of confidence, irritability and anger. A mismatch between the expectations of the individual and that of the organization with regard to role can lead to conflict. An example of this is mentioned later in the section on burnout.

ROLE OVERLOAD

The number of roles that one person has to handle can become too much. Role overload is different to work overload (i.e. having too much work to do overall). The latter can mean there is too much to do in one role. Role overload is to do with variety as well as quantity and an example of this will be presented in the section on burnout.

Readers may wish to write down all the various roles involved in their job. Are there really too many roles for one person to handle? Is it sometimes difficult to perform different roles at the same time (i.e. do some of your roles conflict with each other)?

ROLE UNDERLOAD

This can arise when individuals are given work to do that does not fit with their perception of their capabilities, i.e. they perceive that they can handle a bigger role. This raises the issue of an optimal role for an individual. Too little challenge can be as stressful as too many demands. (For a discussion of this concept, usually referred to as the **inverted U hypothesis**, the reader is referred to, for example, French and Caplan, 1973.)

Handy (1985) suggests that role overload can be reduced by down-grading the importance of some roles and turning in low performance in those areas, in the knowledge that they are less important, and also by an agreed reassignment of role responsibilities and priorities. Role underload can be made easier for the individual by, for example, taking on someone else's role as well as his/her own.

There are many other sources of stress in organizations, including problems relating to career development (e.g. overpromotion, under-promotion), interpersonal relationships with clients, peers and managers, and problems arising from working as part of a team, as well as the organizational structure and climate (e.g. the extent to which people are consulted and involved). An example of the latter is when a group of nurses were told that they would have to rotate between working days and nights and this was not discussed with them until the decision had been made. An additional problem can be conflicting pressures between home and work. The interested reader is referred to, for example, Cooper and Cartwright, 1997, Sutherland and Cooper, 1990 and Vachon, 1988.

REDUCING THE CHANCES OF BECOMING BURNT OUT

> While I was on holiday I was acutely ill in bed with flu. I felt so physically ill it was really quite a struggle even to get myself back but I was back into a full schedule at work the day after I got back and I honoured those commitments. I didn't have any time off sick at all, I just kept going. I was feeling absolutely terrible. About 3 months later I had a weekend when I was just very weepy and I couldn't stop crying and I just realized that I couldn't go into work on the Monday and I virtually slept solidly for a week.

This was part of an account of a worker in a voluntary counselling agency. Over a period of 7 or 8 years she had taken on multiple roles, including administration, training and counselling, and worked long hours including some evenings and weekends. Burnout is described as emotional exhaustion and cynicism towards one's work. Signs can include feeling 'used up' at the end of the working day, not really caring what happens to some clients, a feeling that one is working too hard on the job and generally feeling emotionally drained and frustrated. On a burnout inventory (Maslach and Jackson, 1981), this worker scored very highly on emotional exhaustion, e.g. 'I feel emotionally drained from my work'. Also, on a sources of pressure at work scale (Cushway *et al.*, 1996) she scored highly on workload, lack of resources, client-related difficulties and home–work conflict.

Further quotes from the above account will help to illustrate some of the possible reasons for becoming burnt out.

GOOD ENOUGH ISN'T GOOD ENOUGH

I think I have a sort of perfectionistic streak in me, which in itself is another pressure, that good enough isn't good enough for me. In terms of my objective and the kinds of standards I was setting myself, I wasn't happy to compromise those.

This is an internal source of pressure and the issue will be referred to again in Chapter 3. If our standards are very high and there are times when it is difficult to maintain them, we will probably be tempted to push ourselves even harder at these times. Such self-pressure in the face of being overloaded will undoubtedly increase the likelihood of becoming burnt out.

A SENSE OF ISOLATION

I think what was fairly isolating was, I don't think many people in the organization just realized how many roles I was trying to fulfil.

There was one person in the organization who supported me both in the sense of having a lot of contact and taking some initiatives himself. About a year before I had the crisis of feeling burnt out, he left and there was nobody else who took on quite so active a supportive role. He was quite a loss in terms of a support person.

Pines and Aronson (1988) describe various kinds of support, including technical appreciation, which comes from an expert who gives helpful feedback on your performance and appreciates what you are doing, and emotional challenge, i.e. having someone who can ask questions such as 'Are you pushing yourself too hard and trying to do too much?' Even though this worker was in a generally positive atmosphere and supportive environment, she was lacking individual technical appreciation and emotional challenge, particularly in the year prior to her burnout crisis.

PACE OF CHANGE

In a sense, part of my own exhaustion came from always having a clear next step to go for and not giving myself a rest from the past development.

There was a lot of change. We started as a pilot project and it was an evolving thing. There was change in relation to funding and moving to different premises. All the time there were some changes in terms of recruitment of more volunteers and training. At one point we appointed someone who didn't fit with the general direction of the organization, which was very difficult.

Having to cope with constant change can be very stressful. Someone who can challenge your ways of thinking and working can be helpful (Pines and Aronson, 1988 refer to this as technical challenge).

FACTORS OUTSIDE WORK

Life outside work was affected to the extent that I was so exhausted that everything sort of slowed down.

The relationship of one of my relatives broke up and he came to live with us. I was trying very hard because of the pressure he was under not to betray too much of what was difficult for me. I was having to support him and this was another source of pressure.

Sometimes stress at work can be counterbalanced by having support and interests outside work that help one to 'switch off.' One of the authors once asked several interviewees how they coped with pressure at work and they all responded with an example of an outside interest. Clearly in the case of this worker such 'switching off' was very difficult because of other factors.

POSITIVE FEEDBACK AND APPRECIATION MAY NOT BE ENOUGH

In some ways the positive feedback and appreciation masked the pressure. It did sustain me but it wasn't a complete antidote to all the volume of work or the diversity of the work.

This illustrates the importance of having various types of support. Had this worker been in a more critical or negative environment she might well have burnt out sooner. The positive atmosphere played a part in keeping her going but in itself was not enough to prevent burnout developing.

PREVENTING BURNOUT

Having reviewed some of the factors contributing to this worker's burnout, it would be helpful to summarize some of the possible ways it might have been prevented. If someone tends to be a perfectionist and good enough isn't good enough it may be worth asking questions such as 'Does everything have to be done to the same standard?' An example of this might be, do reports for internal consumption have to be of the same standard as those that will be read by people outside the organization? Another question might be 'In terms of priorities, how important is this piece of work?' A lower priority, less important task could be carried out at a lower standard.

A variety of support mechanisms is important. Just one type of support may not be sufficient. Having technical appreciation and technical and emotional challenge is important as well as having someone to generally listen and support. (This theme will be developed further in Chapter 16.) One nurse made use of peer group support, but twice in a period of 12 years, when he was experiencing crises at work, he was able to turn to a senior nurse manager for support. This access to different kinds of support probably played a role in preventing him from becoming burnt out.

Having activities/interests outside of work that can help one to 'switch off' and maintain a sense of balance can be helpful. One nurse who had experienced a varied and stressful career felt that he had avoided becoming burnt out by maintaining various outside interests, by making time to do things with his family and by being very disciplined with himself: 'You've got to say, "Right, this is it now, no more today. I've done 10 hours, you're not having any more of my time. It's a 24-hour service, you must find somebody else." '

Miller (1991) reviews occupational burnout and morbidity generally and in relation to HIV/AIDS carers. Examples of suggestions for the prevention of burnout generally include: orientation programmes for new staff; developing and promoting a strong professional philosophy and ethos – a team spirit; training in recognizing distress; modifying roles and workloads; more participation in decision making; individuals having realistic expectations; encouraging personal responsibility for health, including eating, exercise and taking time off when sick.

Suggestions for prevention of burnout in HIV/AIDS workers include psychological preparation for AIDS work before working on the wards, backed up with opportunities for regular psychological referral, and also training of physicians, nurses and others to incorporate more realistic expectations about their own capabilities and responses to 'failures' of treatment.

Other suggestions for preventing burnout made by Wright (1993) include on-going education as a means of eliminating feelings of being professionally inadequate and giving stimulation and more confidence; also looking at alternatives and thinking about a move or change and discussing your role and direction in your career with a colleague.

COPING GENERALLY WITH THE STRESS OF CHANGE

Hopson (1981), whose model of change was described in Chapter 1, makes various suggestions for managing change. His view is that there are two tasks that need to be performed:

- **management of strain**, i.e. to cope in such a way that one can engage the problems caused by the transition;
- **cognitive coping tasks**, i.e. adjusting by making decisions about the appropriateness of new and old behaviours.

He describes a useful coping skills questionnaire the first section of which is about knowing yourself. This is probably one of the most important factors in coping with transitions and one of the authors has adapted some of the questions for working with people experiencing change, e.g. those preparing for retirement. Questions that people are asked to consider include:

- Can I think of two of my strengths?
- Can I think of two of my weaknesses?
- Do I know other people's view of me (and is this view accurate)?
- Do I easily let go of old situations?
- If I feel under stress, do I know what I can do to help myself?
- Do I find it easy to express my feelings?
- Do I take initiatives or sit back and wait for things to happen?

The last question is particularly interesting. Some people coming up to retirement say that they fear they may find it difficult to get up in the morning if they do not have the structure of a working day. They may just laze around doing nothing in particular. Their task then becomes shifting to being more proactive, perhaps beginning to explore alternatives to work that give their lives some structure.

The worker whose experience was described in the section on burnout recognized that she needed a change of gear and negotiated with her organization to have a year's sabbatical. 'I felt that I'd got to take control of it, rather than be controlled by it, and actually make a choice rather than perpetuating what had gone on.' She decided that she was going to make something happen and look for something else. This proactive stance was experienced as a liberating feeling: 'I don't have to stay in this situation, I'm not trapped in this for ever.'

Being aware of strengths and weaknesses can open up the possibility of dealing with change more constructively. For example, some people may take on board more and more work because they want to appear helpful and find it difficult to say no. Admitting to oneself that this is the reason for becoming overburdened may give the courage to start saying no, or some new skills may need to be practised in the area of being more assertive.

For some people, their strength may be that they can stand back from a situation, think clearly about priorities and put other things on the back-burner. This strength can be used to help them and colleagues to cope better with change.

Another important aspect of coping with change is to think about other important changes or events in your life. Questions to ask might include the following:

- Do I remember how I felt when it happened?
- Was I prepared for it?
- Was there anyone to talk to/anyone to help?
- What did I do to help myself get through that experience?
- What would I have done differently to make it easier?
- What have I learnt about myself as a result of that experience?

If, in the face of past change, people have stuck their heads in the sand and refused to accept it, this has probably made them less able to cope with the tasks facing them in their new situation. Some staff in a hospital that has been under the threat of closure for many years commented to one of the authors, 'They've been talking about closure for so long, I can't believe it will ever happen.' Questioning whether this way of dealing with change was helpful in the past and what might have been done differently opens up the possibility of changing one's approach in a more constructive direction. This could involve asking questions such as 'What if the worst did happen, if this place did close?' and 'Maybe I ought to give some thought to possible alternatives?'

Some people may have found it helpful in the past to sound out ideas with other people, to use them as a sounding board or to take some time out to reflect on their new situation. If this approach was helpful in the past it may be useful in coping with a current transition.

Generally it can be helpful to consider how personal characteristics may help or hinder one's ability to cope with change. The problem of saying no was mentioned above and, as already described, the worker in the section on burnout had problems with being a perfectionist. Friedman and Rosenman (1974) describe the Type A personality as some-body who is hard-driving, aggressive and finds it difficult to listen and be patient (e.g. would become very frustrated in a queue or traffic jam). Such behaviour is likely to be maladaptive in coping with change; indeed it places individuals at higher risk of having a heart attack. There are various cognitive and behavioural strategies that might help to reduce such behaviour, e.g. learning to relax and telling oneself to slow down, that it doesn't matter if one is held up for a while.

Kobasa (1982) described the attitude of hardiness, which helps people to cope better with stress. It consists of a sense of challenge, commitment and control. Stress-hardy people tend to see a challenge where others would see a threat; they are involved, for instance with work, family and friends, and see these involvements as interesting and meaningful. A sense of control comes from having skills and self-confidence and the belief that one can cope with stress. For many situations this kind of attitude can act as a buffer against stress. Another personal characteristic that can affect ability to cope with the stress of change is locus of control (Rotter, 1966). People with an internal locus of control tend to feel they can influence events whereas those with an external locus are more likely to put things down to, for instance, fate.

MAINTAINING A SENSE OF SELF-WORTH AND VALUE

The reader may wish to reflect how many times recently somebody at work has said 'Thank you' or 'You've done a good job there' or 'I really appreciate you taking on that task' or any similar comment. Unfortunately, some people only hear from their manager when something has gone wrong or a complaint has been made. One nurse manager reported that the way conflicts were resolved in his organization was a source of pressure and that sometimes there was a lack of exoneration when unjustified complaints were made. This made nurses feel angry.

The insidious nature of feeling undervalued is captured in the following comment from a nurse ward manager:

> On a bad day you can feel pretty undervalued and neglected. It's as though the system is changing almost to the point that it's trying to catch you out and trying to make you keep up to speed. Asking more and more out of fewer and fewer people. So it's very difficult, if I'm honest, to keep a measure of self-worth. This if you're not careful can spread to other staff as well. They begin to feel that they are just a number and they're not appreciated any more.

Some nurses realize the importance of acknowledging their colleagues' efforts. For example, a ward manager always thanks his staff as they go off duty and a staff nurse always gives students 5 minutes at the end of a shift to talk about their day and say thank you.

For people who enter the helping professions, the initial motivation is often to do something useful, to help others, and this will probably be one of their values. Therefore, feedback from the recipients of help can be an important source of self-esteem. This was illustrated in the third quote at the beginning of this chapter, in which a caregiver received positive comments from a patient with AIDS. Below are two further examples of such feedback received from people in the counselling professions:

> I wish to offer my sincere thanks for your kindness and consideration and to say I derived much help from my meetings with you. The dreadful sorrow I had over my son's death has now reached a stage where I'm sure I can cope and I think will ease with the passage of time.

> I had been seeing this client for about a year and I suggested a finishing date. She was angry and upset about it and in the end did not come to the last part of the therapy. I had doubts about whether I had been right to finish with her; had it been damaging, had it negated any therapeutic gains? More than a year later I received a letter from this client enclosing a photo of her new baby, for her a very significant event which had been talked about a lot in therapy. It emerged from the letter that she was doing quite well and I felt touched by her making this contact with me and felt that therapy had after all been important for her.

It may be that such feedback does not necessarily just reflect a therapist's skill and competence. The clients may, for example, have been grateful for someone to listen and take them seriously. The problem of social desirability (telling you what they think you want to hear) can operate with solicited feedback. However, this is less likely with the above examples of unsolicited feedback. As one therapist put it, 'It is good when clients show appreciation, especially if this seems "real" rather than just polite'. Positive appraisal can be very gratifying, particularly if one doubted the effectiveness of one's help, as in the second example above.

A psychologist who worked with children was made starkly aware of the value of feedback when she moved from a job in education in which it was plentiful to one in health care in which it was minimal:

> In my previous job I received positive feedback on almost a daily basis. It came from almost everyone I worked with – parents, school staff and colleagues. I was frequently thanked for 'everything that I had done'. I also received a number of overwhelming comments, e.g. one teacher stood up in the staff room and said that I was the best psychologist she'd known in 30 years of teaching. I was frequently made aware that I was discussed by headteachers because they valued my work. I was welcomed with open arms everywhere I went, it was wonderful.

> In my current job I find that there is very little positive feedback. Occasionally children write to me and I get small gifts. I really appreciate it when families come back to tell me that everything is OK and 'thank you' but it doesn't happen that often.

This psychologist went on to explain how she missed a structured staff appraisal scheme, in which there were opportunities for appraisals from both peers and more senior staff. It helped her to take stock of good work and achievements. Another way of receiving positive feedback is to give it to oneself: if you have done a good job, then give yourself a pat on the back (e.g. 'I did a good job there, it was worth all the effort'). This worker made the interesting point that, though she gave herself a pat on the back a lot in her old job she seldom did in her current job because she rarely got a pat on the back from anyone else. It is probably very difficult to generate internal 'well dones' in the absence of external validation that you have done a good job.

Larson (1993) refers to this connection between external and internal reinforcement in his 'feel good – do good' theory of helping. Positive feedback or events can ignite a 'glow of goodwill' that leads to helping and a concern for the well-being of others. Once helping begins, it can then be intrinsically reinforcing and it can make you feel better. Another factor that may affect giving oneself a pat on the back is locus of control, mentioned in the previous section. By contrasting her experience in the two jobs, the above psychologist was of the opinion that people don't work as well or achieve as much when they don't feel valued.

A similar contrast was reported by a nurse who used to be a teacher. Nobody ever told her she was doing a good job as a nurse but she felt very valued as a teacher: 'I got a lot of feedback from the headmistress. I was promoted in my second year because she said I was doing a good job and she wanted me to stay there. I felt really valued, I felt great.'

Meetings and discussions with colleagues who work in similar ways to oneself and share the same approach and values can help to maintain a sense of value. Pines and Aronson (1988) speak of this as shared social reality. Some workers place a lot of importance on feeling valued by professional colleagues in the same team.

Some organizations set up systems that aim to get people more involved in decision making and thus provide a forum for valuing their contribution more. One such approach is the use of quality circles or voluntary improvement teams. These originated in Japan and the United States and were introduced into British health care in the 1980s (see, for instance, Spall et al., 1992). Essentially, they are small problem-solving groups where staff get together on a regular basis to analyse and produce solutions to work-related problems. Their most important feature is that, set up properly, they have the full commitment and backing of senior management, who take an interest in the work of the groups and provide quick support for the implementation of good problem solutions when necessary. The most enlightened chief executives and senior managers will encourage the groups by occasionally going to talk to them about their progress. It can be a boost to morale when a senior member of the organization takes the time to talk to you about your work.

In this chapter we have considered the environment in which many professional helpers have to work. Understanding the factors in organizations that can lead to stress and burnout increases the chances of preventing these consequences. Being aware of how one's personal characteristics and usual ways of coping with change can help or hinder also opens up the possibility of coping better with a stressful environment. We have also considered the important and often neglected area of maintaining a sense of value. If this chapter has given you ideas on how to cope better with a changing, uncertain environment and at the same time maintain a sense of self-worth, then you will be better prepared to work effectively with people experiencing various forms of loss.

Being professional 3

Nurses struggled between expressing their sad feelings and knowing such emotional expression contradicted the expectations for professional behaviour.

Davies et al., 1996 –
a study of paediatric nurses

When people have died, I've cried with the relatives and I don't think really it's unprofessional ... but I think a general nurse would think that unprofessional.

Psychiatric nurse

You say expected empty things
You speak in pious tones
You call on God to heal the man
When
What you really say is,
'Get me out of here'.

Autton, 1969

The concept of a professional helper encompasses many strands. These include:

- a set of expectations the helpers have of themselves;
- expectations of the helper's clients;
- expectations that different helpers have of each other.

Problems may arise if some of these expectations are too high or there is a discrepancy between helper expectations of self and those of others. In this chapter we aim to consider how the notion of being professional may be both helpful and unhelpful in the ways in which it can affect the provision of good quality helping and care. Firstly, though, we need to discuss what it means to be a professional.

THE CONCEPT OF BEING A PROFESSIONAL

Potter and Perry (1993) offer a definition of being professional in the context of nursing. They write, 'When we say a person acts "professionally", for example, we imply that the person is conscientious in actions, knowledgeable in the subject, and responsible to self and others.' These authors also quote Etzioni (1961), who refers to the following extended definition of what it means to be a professional:

- A profession requires an extended education of its members, as well as a basic liberal foundation.
- A profession has a theoretical body of knowledge, leading to defined skills, abilities and norms.
- A profession provides a specific service.
- Members of a profession have autonomy in decision making and practice.
- The profession as a whole has a code of ethics for practice.

Williams (1993), in discussing the characteristics of being professional, points out that it also involves tests of the competence of members of the profession and the provision of altruistic service. This latter ideal (with which many may enter the caring professions) may not always be achievable, especially if one is feeling undervalued or under high levels of stress.

As mentioned above, Etzioni (1961) suggests that a profession provides a specific service. This implies that the members of that profession are quite clear as to the boundaries to the work they have to do as members of that profession. Is that always true of caring professions? Certainly, the nursing profession is in a state of flux as to exactly where their role ends and that of the doctor begins.

An instance of this question of role demarcation came to the attention of the British Press in 1996. It was reported that a senior theatre sister had carried out an appendectomy under the supervision of an experienced surgeon. There was no question as to the quality of the work performed by the nurse. Questions were raised, though, that had to do with going beyond the bounds of her demarcated area of responsibility. Had she overstepped the bounds of being professional? In the UK there is also debate at the time of writing within the medical profession as to whether nurses should be allowed to prescribe drugs on a limited basis.

The issue of the boundary of professional responsibility also touches on the area of competence. One of the aspects of being professional referred to previously is having a theoretical body of knowledge that leads to defined skills, abilities and norms. This is probably commonly accepted by various professions. However, there can be a conflict when people outside the profession fail to acknowledge these things as important characteristics of that profession. Hugman (1991) speaks of the public's perception of nurses, for instance, as being carers and nurturers rather than competent professionals.

CONFLICT OF RESPONSIBILITIES CAN AFFECT CARE

As professionals where does our responsibility lie? Is it to the organization that we work for, to the clients or patients we serve or to ourselves? Perhaps the answer is to all three. A Health Authority spokesman quoted on British television in 1994 said that the first responsibility of doctors was to the organization. The response of the doctors was one of outrage that the needs of the patients were not considered paramount.

A psychiatric nursing sister spoke of the problems with management *vis-à-vis* her not being able to give a professional service. She said:

I expect to be able to give the care that I should be giving and I'm not. And that's what frustrates me. I'm not giving what I should be giving ... that I can't give the care that I want to give. And I do get very angry at meetings and I do try and fight ... and I've won in some cases but it's just been one long fight with management. And I get to the point where I'm sick of it. I'm sick of the fighting.

A nurse therapist has spoken of the conflict she has between the social work fundholder looking for time-limited counselling and the therapist's view, as provider, that the client needed more time to explore her difficulties.

These examples of conflict between purchasers or managers of services and the helping professionals providing the services point to the need to take a wider perspective on professional care. If as helping professionals we do not have broader support to enable us to do the job, then it may not be possible to reach either our own expectations of ourselves or the expectations of others. Responsibility is a two-way process: while we may have a responsibility to the organization we work for, it also needs to enable helpers to provide professional care. A specific example of conflict that may affect care is the organizational need to monitor and record and the amount of time this takes, which detracts from the time available for face-to-face help to clients.

A social worker when asked what he thought it meant to be professional said, 'Being professional means putting the needs of other people first, foremost and totally, without allowing one's own needs to prejudice or bias.' Can one really separate the client's needs from the professional's? A professional who gives no heed to his or her own needs increases the risk of becoming burnt out. When this happens, are the client's needs being put first if the social worker is unable to work, or is working less effectively? Even at an earlier stage than full burnout, a professional who is overtired is unlikely to provide the best service to clients.

Another example of potential conflict between a client's needs and those of the professional helper relates to the issue of confidentiality. Many helpers gain a measure of support by talking about the events of the day or week to friends or family. But does such conversation breach confidentiality? For example, can we really be sure that the person we are talking to does not know the client we are speaking about? If we are talking to colleagues or friends, perhaps informally in a public house or restaurant, can we be sure that we are not being overheard by someone who might know the person we are discussing? The offloading of the stress involved in caring is clearly important for the professional helper. However, confidentiality is also very important, as it enables clients to maintain trust, which is necessary for the opening up of innermost concerns.

It could be argued that, when bad news is broken to a relative rather than the patient, this is a breach of confidentiality. This situation probably arises because of a conflict of needs. The patient may need to know the diagnosis and prognosis but the professional helper may need to be protected from an angry response or from being confronted directly with failure and his or her own mortality (see Chapter 11).

Being aware of how conflict of responsibilities can affect care can be helpful. It modifies any simplistic notion that we should provide a high quality of professional care and that if we don't it is a reflection of weakness in ourselves.

THE EFFECTS OF UNREALISTIC EXPECTATIONS

For some people, expectations about being a professional are unrealistic. When a group of psychiatric nurses were asked what it meant to be professional, responses included comments like, 'being godlike' and 'being all things to all men'. In another context, a group of teachers comments about being professional in working with children experiencing loss included, 'give love and friendship' and 'provide whatever the child seems to need from me'. Subscribing to such high ideals is setting oneself up for failure. Even if they could be achieved some of the time, it would not be possible to maintain such idealistic care. The consequent failure to achieve these expected goals is likely to lead to increased dissatisfaction and stress for these professional helpers.

Sometimes expectations may exert an effect even though they are not explicitly stated or discussed. In the study by Davies *et al.* (1996) quoted at the beginning of this chapter the implicit expectations among nurses caring for dying children included that they should be cheerful at all times and not cry when on duty; also that they should be strong for the patient and other nurses and refrain from getting emotionally involved with patients and their families. In this study nurses who 'went along' with these expectations and did not acknowledge their need to express sad emotions were less able to manage their distress.

Unrealistic expectations are not confined to professionals. Sometimes they come from members of the public and are reflected in the way they perceive professionals. On an anecdotal level, it is common to hear a phrase like 'It's marvellous what they can do nowadays' among lay people discussing medicine and an individual who is very ill. Spiegel (1977), writing of doctors in the context of breaking bad news, talks of the views of those who are the recipients of the doctor's skill. 'He possesses authority and power. In addition, there is not only the hope and confidence in his ability to heal on the part of the patient and his family but also the expectations in his magical omnipotence and infallibility.' Doctors who become aware of such views may feel under a lot of pressure to fulfil these expectations, even though they realize the impossibility of always meeting them.

Perhaps the most helpful question to ask, if there are unrealistic expectations around, is 'Where do they come from?' If they are self-imposed, perhaps we could try to lower them a little. If they come from clients, we could try not to collude with them while at the same time aiming to maintain a degree of hope. When unrealistic expectations originate from peers or managers, open communication about the issue is clearly a good starting point.

EXUDING CONFIDENCE AND FEELING VULNERABLE

At particularly anxious and vulnerable times in their lives, it is undoubtedly important for clients to feel confident in their professional helpers. Hence an air of confidence in the latter should be helpful. An analogy here may be instructive. When we take our car to the garage for repair we want to know that the mechanics are competent at their job. In finding a garage we take into account such things as whether it is on one of the motoring organizations' approved lists. We may ask others who have had their cars serviced or repaired at garages in the area for their recommendation.

On an unconscious level, though, we are reassured by the apparent honesty of the mechanic's face. The overalls being worn and the impressive array of tools on the garage walls may also help to create an impression of competence. In our thinking about hospitals, the same process is likely to be at work. The consultants and the firms that work under them gain in reputation within the area and sometimes nationally. Our anxieties are also allayed by the sight of doctors in their white coats decorated with a stethoscope that is either around their necks or half out of a pocket. We are equally helped by the nurses' uniform and the regimented positioning of hospital beds. Even the consultants' failure to wear the white coat of other doctors is somehow reassuring. The lack of uniform seems to be saying that they have reached such a position that they do not need to wear a badge of competence any more.

Goffman (1959) wrote about how people relate to each other in their daily business. His contention is that we rarely play ourselves when we are in conversation with others. Rather, we play a role that is appropriate for the situation we are in. He writes:

> When an individual plays a part he implicitly requests his observers to take seriously the impression that is fostered before them. They are asked to believe that the character they see actually possesses the attributes he appears to possess, that the tasks he performs will have the consequences that are implicitly claimed for it, and that, in general, matters are what they appear to be.

Clearly, giving the impression that one is confident and competent in one's professional role may be very important.

Autton (1969), in his handbook for hospital chaplains quoted at the beginning of this chapter, suggests that a professional exterior is as important for professionals as for their clients. He also suggests that it is adopted by the professional to hide a real weakness. He writes, 'The clergyman's unction, the physician's wise mien . . . are all of them indications of signs of weakness resorted to in order to cover the poverty of the real self.'

This brings us to the other side of the coin to exuding confidence, namely that underlying it there may be a feeling of vulnerability. Things may not be as they seem. One of the authors has a clear memory of struggling with his vocation when deciding to enter the pastoral ministry. One of the reasons he did not want to pursue his application was the thought that once ordained he would be put on a pedestal by church members and expected to remain balancing on it. The thought of having to live up to standards that other mortals were not expected to maintain was very daunting to him.

A psychiatric nurse said, 'I think people are vulnerable, I think we all are. Everybody thinks that doctors are so right and people go along with what they say, and it doesn't always follow, does it?' A general trained nurse expressed a similar misgiving about the role of nurses. 'I think that most people have this professional image in their heads of what a nurse is. We're supposed to be kind, we're supposed to be caring, we're supposed to be supportive. We're never supposed to show that we're upset, and our emotions are always supposed to be in check. I think it's almost a false image.'

We will discuss in Chapter 4 how professional helpers may be affected by loss at work and how personal loss may impinge on work. Accepting our own vulnerability is an important first step on the road to effective helping. Having accepted this, it highlights the need for support mechanisms, which will be discussed specifically in Chapter 16.

CLINICAL DETACHMENT VERSUS THE ACKNOWLEDGEMENT OF FEELINGS

The notion of clinical detachment being helpful seems to be related to a concern that the opposite, overinvolvement, is detrimental. If one becomes overinvolved, then one's judgement and objectivity may be impaired and decisions may not be in the best interest of the client. When a professional is on duty, the needs of the client should be considered primary. This is reflected by Burnard and Chapman (1993) in their statement, 'The attitude of the professional towards the client is one of service on an individual basis, the client's needs being placed before those of the professional.' This approach is illustrated in the following comment from a nurse: 'I hope I didn't reflect my own emotional trauma on them [patients] and then as soon as I left work it used to hit me again. But I made a point of saying to myself, "You've got to work and not to inflict your stress on them." '

The problem with clinical detachment is that it can be associated with a denial of the importance of acknowledging feelings. McMahon and Pearson (1991) write: 'In the past the nurse was expected to maintain a relationship that did not encourage the expression of feelings by the patient or the nurse. This was justified on the grounds that it was not "professional" to do so and that nurses could not cope with the stress that would ensue.' Burnard and Chapman (1993) write in a similar vein when they say, 'In nursing it is often far easier (and sometimes encouraged) either to ignore or to rationalize feelings as they occur in day-to-day practice and even to pretend that they simply do not exist. This is evident in the image of the nurse as an implacable, objective carer who has somehow learned to detach herself from emotion.' An illustration of this philosophy was provided by a nurse tutor with a special interest in terminal care, who spoke of her training 20 years ago. She recalled sitting with a dying patient and becoming upset when the patient died. Her superiors made it very clear that her display of emotion was unacceptable and she seriously considered giving up her career at that point. Fortunately, she continued to nurse.

A social worker also reflected this attitude when she said to the authors, 'I've always been taught about this "stiff upper lip". That you never show your feelings to the public or to clients.' A general trained nurse had the same experience. She told us, 'I was 17, I'm 53 next month and I was always taught to be professional and not to – I was originally taught not to have any feelings and not to show emotions.' She went on to say, 'I realize now that it's quite acceptable to get uptight and upset and what have you, but I've always – never backed away. If I haven't liked nursing a patient, or been upset, I've always gone on. That's because of the way I've been trained.'

Burnard and Chapman (1993) discuss how the old view of being detached is inappropriate and that a level of involvement is important in providing effective care.

> The nurse has to return to the role of a nurse using the knowledge gained to enhance the care given. This does require that the nurse becomes involved with the patient, an activity frequently frowned on in the past and still regarded with suspicion by many as being 'unprofessional'. What is unprofessional is an impersonal approach which results in all patients being treated as if they are identical, which is clearly not the case.

These authors also go on to say that the nature of nursing is very distressing, and that nurses are called upon to treat people in very difficult circumstances. Given this, the whole question of the display of feelings needs to be addressed in both clinical and educational circles. 'The profession cannot afford to carry on as though nurses were somehow detached emotionally. Human suffering always calls for involvement, and involvement in the human condition always includes feelings. To ignore the domain of feelings in nurses is to ignore an important part of what it means to be a human being.' These comments about nurses clearly have relevance to doctors and other health-care professionals.

We are not protected from fears, anxieties and other normal emotional reactions associated with loss by being in the role of professional helper. Lugton (1987) makes this point in the context of hospice care and also reiterates the importance of acknowledging such feelings.

> I believe that it is important to have some insight into our feelings and to be able to acknowledge when we are upset, rather than giving the appearance to colleagues and to patients that nothing ever troubles us. Being professional and retaining the ability to support others, does not in my experience, mean being invulnerable to feeling sad, or on occasions, angry.

In this chapter we have discussed how views and expectations about being professional can impinge on the helping and care that is provided. An experienced, well-informed professional can present a confident image to clients. However, there are various factors that can undermine effective helping, including a conflict of responsibilities, unrealistic expectations and a failure to acknowledge one's feelings and vulnerability. In order to further raise awareness of these issues, the reader may wish to address the following questions.

Thoughts on how 'being professional' might affect my helping

- What do I expect of myself as a professional?
- What do I think that my clients expect of me as a professional?
- Are the expectations in the first two questions realistic?
- Is there a discrepancy between the expectations others have of me and those I have of myself? If there is, how do I deal with it?
- Am I clear about my own needs as a professional helper, as well as the needs of my clients?
- How do I balance the conflicting responsibilities to the organization I work for, to my clients and to myself?
- Am I confident that I, and those I work with, are clear as to the boundaries of my responsibility as a professional?
- Am I able to acknowledge difficult feelings or do I prefer to maintain a degree of detachment?
- How are my own needs as a professional helper met?
- Specifically, do I meet my own needs to offload in ways that don't compromise client confidentiality?

Experienced loss – can it affect our work?

4

Grief is a common reaction of professionals to the suffering, loss and death of patients. Working in a professional role does not protect individuals from the emotional impact of death related experiences.

Cook and Oltjenbruns, 1989

This lady had a mastectomy. She was my age. What could I say when I was told that there was no hope ... the cancer had spread ... She had little kids too! I broke down and cried.

Nurse quoted in Lerea and LiMauro, 1982

One boy's mum died this year. I felt his hurt very personally and was determined to give him whatever he needed to help him cope.

Primary School Teacher

I work on a women's ward and I haven't spoken to my mother in 6 years. I think I feel very envious of some of the mother–daughter relationships I see on the ward.

General Nurse

This chapter addresses the ways in which experienced loss can affect the work of a professional helper. Such losses may be personal and occur outside of work or be related to the work situation. Personal loss may be actual events such as the death of a relative or 'non-events', i.e. loss in the form of something that ought to happen but never occurs; an example of this form of loss is not being able to have children. Some professionals may be at risk of the effects of accumulated loss at work. They may barely have had time to think about or work through previous losses when another one comes along. It will be argued that loss is an area where it is difficult to neatly separate off our personal and professional lives. Illustrations of the interaction between personal and working lives will be presented. This will include the situation when there are similarities between the client's experience and our own and the problem of identification.

Whatever form of loss is experienced, it could affect work with clients in either a positive or negative way. One of the factors which will determine the impact on work is the extent to which the loss has been adjusted to or worked through.

WORK-RELATED GRIEF

Lerea and LiMauro (1982) compared grief reactions among nursing staff in a general hospital and a skilled nursing facility for older patients. Overall 98% of general hospital staff and 63% of nursing facility staff answered yes to the question 'Have you ever grieved in response to your patients' physical/emotional condition?' In both settings, psychological symptoms of grief exceeded physical reactions. The most common psychological reactions, mentioned by 50% or more of their sample of 100 respondents, were:

- thinking or talking about the patient;
- feelings of helplessness;
- crying or despondency;
- disbelief or shock;
- difficulty concentrating;
- anger towards others.

Of particular interest was their finding that, more than one month after the critical incident, bereavement reactions continued to be felt by 50% of the general hospital staff and 38% of the specialist nursing facility staff. This is relevant to the issue of the effects of a build-up of losses. If several losses occur close together there may be problems with finding the time and space to grieve for each loss (see Accumulated loss, below).

Other findings included the observation that cancer was the diagnosis that elicited grief most often among respondents in both settings. Also, there was no significant difference between the grief reactions of nurses and nurse aides. Possible explanations offered for differences between staff reactions in the two settings included whether the death was timely or anticipated and the extent to which there were expectations of improvement.

SOME FACTORS THAT CAN AFFECT GRIEF AT WORK

AGE

The death of an older person can be less stressful because it is 'on time' – a natural, predictable occurrence of later life. The loss of a younger person, by contrast, may be more stressful because the event is what Neugarten (1972) refers to as 'off time'.

Cook and Oltjenbruns (1989) followed up the effects of a sudden infant death syndrome (SIDS) death on a hospital team involved in the infant's care. Reactions included shock, disbelief and guilt. The staff member who had spent most time with the SIDS victim was initially fearful of handling other infants and reported frequent crying, appetite problems and bad dreams associated with the death.

The death of an older person may be viewed as timely and sometimes as a blessing because it is a relief from suffering. Lerea and LiMauro (1982) quote a nurse working with older people: 'Mr L lived at — convalescent centre for more than 7 years. He was such a kind, dignified man. I watched him go down all that time . . . unable to feed himself, incontinent, confused. When he died, it was like I lost my own father. I grieved but I was also relieved.'

SUDDEN/UNEXPECTED DEATH

A sudden and unexpected death, as in the sudden infant death described above, typically leads to more difficult grief. There is no time for anticipatory grieving and there may be issues concerning whether the death was preventable.

Suicide is an example of sudden death. If this occurs in hospital, staff may experience overwhelming guilt for failure to prevent the death. Failure to resolve this and other grief reactions may affect future care of other patients at risk of committing suicide (Benner, 1989).

RELATIONSHIP WITH PATIENT

As in the case of the nurse caring for Mr L above, staff caring for patients in long-stay contexts have a considerable time, sometimes years, to form a relationship with them. Sometimes staff may take on the role of surrogate griever in the absence of family support for the dying (Fulton, 1979). This involves acting as a substitute for family members and experiencing some of the associated grief. Grieving is likely to be more difficult than if a nurse is working in an acute medical setting, where patients may only be on the unit for a short period.

On an intensive care unit it is more difficult for a nurse to care for someone who enters the unit in an alert state and then deteriorates (Swanson and Swanson, 1977). The longer the patient is alert and able to communicate, the stronger the staff reaction will be if the patient dies. At the other extreme, caring for someone who enters the unit in a comatose state leads to less grief following the patient's death because there is not really any opportunity for emotional involvement.

PERCEPTIONS OF A GOOD DEATH

Saunders and Valente (1994) reported on some questionnaire findings from over 300 oncology and hospice nurses who had attended their bereavement workshops. Most nurses reported that they felt they managed their grief effectively if they helped the patient to die a **good death**. The factors associated with a good death included the following:

- The nurse had relieved the patient's distress and symptoms (to the extent allowed by current knowledge and technology).
- Patients had the opportunity to complete tasks related to their important relationships.
- The nurse believed that he or she had delivered the best quality of care possible for the patient.

Nurses were proud of managing symptoms and facilitating family communication and this comforted them in their own grief. If they had not been able to help a patient die a good death or when they were off duty when the patient died, their grief was reported to be more difficult. Terms such as 'more complicated', 'difficult', 'painful' and 'distressing' were used. Perceptions of a good death will be discussed again in Chapter 8.

CONSTRUCTIVE USE OF EXPERIENCED LOSS

The relationship between personal loss and performance of one's job can be viewed as a balancing act. Guitarist Eric Clapton wrote a song following the death of his son in 1991. Commenting on his performance of the song he says:

> On occasions it's been close to where I would choke and not be able to do it ... but then what would happen? We'd have to stop and it would get mawkish and embarrassing. At the same time to back off and pretend that it's about nothing and just play it as if it's a song that had no meaning would be pointless, so there's a thin line you have to tread, somewhere in the middle.
>
> Roberty, 1995

Similarly, for professional helpers, who have experienced personal loss, to carry out their work as if the personal loss didn't matter and had no relevance would be denying its significance. At the other extreme the personal loss may interfere with the ability to do the job. Ideally, one should be able to use personal experience to help others in loss situations (as Eric Clapton's song, 'Tears in Heaven', may well have done – the authors are aware of one couple who played it at their child's funeral). Giving such help will not be possible if the personal loss is regarded as irrelevant or if one is overwhelmed by it.

SOME POSITIVE EFFECTS OF EXPERIENCED LOSS

People who experience life-threatening illness or traumatic events often report changed priorities: for instance, material things become less important and more emphasis is placed on relationships. Tedeschi and Calhoun (1995) reviewed several studies that indicate a changed philosophy of life; for example, in women who had made changes since their cancer was discovered 60% talked of positive changes in priorities, such as taking life easier and enjoying it more (Taylor *et al.*, 1984). Also, 94% of the survivors of a cruise ship disaster said that they no longer took life for granted and 71% reported that they now lived each day to the fullest (Joseph *et al.*, 1993).

Similar changes in their attitude to life can occur for professional workers as a direct consequence of their work. A hospice worker reported the following philosophy change to one of the authors after a few years of working with dying patients:

> I feel that life is like a light bulb. I think we think it's strong and it's safe and it burns brightly and it will go on. But if you look at the filament, it is so fragile that it can go any minute. And that's how I feel about life, that we really do take it so much for granted and it can go, just like that.

Such experience confronts us with our own mortality and makes it difficult to maintain a sense of invulnerability. This worker also described learning to respect others' views, not to be intolerant and to cherish people. In addition nature took on a much sharper meaning: 'You notice the sky and the changes in the season matter. This is most probably the only place where you can come and we have an hour's discussion on the tree outside.'

An experienced hospice nurse described several examples of how work has affected her attitude to life: 'I think as you get older in this work you only live for this day because nobody knows what's round the corner. Tomorrow is another day. And its made me more accepting.' When talking of what she had learnt from dying people and their relatives, she reported, 'You learn to be more tolerant, more tolerant of your own family and more tolerant of life and other people and you don't prejudge people the same. And you shouldn't bear grudges, things like that, because life is too short.'

For this nurse an important insight was gained from a patient who noted that there is something good in each person. Sometimes you have to search for it but there is something there. This philosophy helped her to have empathy with a wide range of patients. She commented, for example, that some of the kindest people weren't the most intelligent or articulate and that it had been an enriching experience to know them.

Professional helpers can also use their personal experience to enhance the quality of their work. Klass (1995) describes how a clergyman's dream of his dead son led to a renewed commitment:

> There he was – that lanky 17-year-old whose life I loved better than my own. He looked deeply into my eyes and with a grin on his face, the way he used to do when he was 'buttering me up'. Not a word was spoken, but everything was said that needed to be said for my turning point to come.

This clergyman went on to report a renewed faith. His pain and loss were not to be the end of life but a beginning – 'a beginning to a more compassionate life of quality and caring'.

A general nurse described to one of the authors how the death of her husband's ex-wife affected her:

> She went through an awful lot and showed courage all the way through her cancer. That helped me to understand what patients must be going through. She always believed in the power of the mind. I think I've transferred that to patients with cancer; I encourage them not to give in. So although we never got on, I think she left me with an inheritance and a respect that I didn't know was there until after she died.

Clearly this personal experience helped this nurse to empathize with and work more effectively with patients with cancer.

A hospice nurse, who had two sisters, gained insight into how the death of an only child can affect a parent when her sister-in-law died. The mother of her sister-in-law was very angry that her only daughter had died. Comparisons were made with the hospice nurse's mother, who had three healthy, living daughters. The effect on this nurse's work was revealed in her statement: 'I try now and put a better understanding to our patients' relatives who have got only children. I think I understand them a bit more.' She also referred to the effect of the untimeliness of her sister-in-law's death from a parent's point of view. You expect your children to go on after you and it made her more aware that she should enjoy her own children and family. This example illustrates the point made at the beginning of this chapter. This nurse's experience affected her attitudes at work and in her personal life. Being open to learning, she was not neatly separating off her professional and private lives.

AWARENESS OF THE NEGATIVE EFFECTS OF
EXPERIENCED LOSS CAN HELP

Larson (1993) describes a useful metaphor for thinking about helping – the helper's pit. The person you are helping is in a pit and you are on

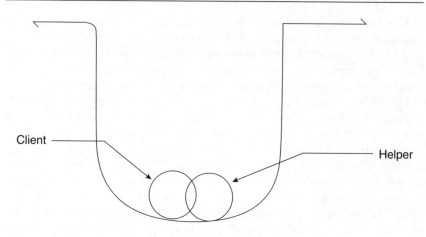

Figure 4.1   In the Helper's Pit (enmeshed/overinvolved).

the edge of the pit. If you identify too closely with this person's problems, you fall into the pit with them. This is the enmeshed or overinvolved position, illustrated in Figure 4.1.

To extend the metaphor, it is possible for a helper to show empathy or sympathy by staying on the edge of the pit or by holding on to a branch and reaching in. This is the 'present but separate' position.

The experience of a social worker working with bereaved people illustrates the problem of overinvolvement:

> I want to mop up their tears and make everything all right again and you can't. So sometimes I get enmeshed in their grief as well and feel as helpless and hopeless as they do ... And I feel like I'm a little beetle on my back with my legs in the air, struggling to get the right way up, and so is the client.

In terms of the pit analogy, for this worker the branch has broken and she has fallen in with the client.

EXTRAPOLATING FROM PERSONAL EXPERIENCE MAY NOT BE HELPFUL

The example given above demonstrates how it can be difficult to work with the bereaved who get stuck and can't move on. The same worker commented on this in relation to her own experience: 'I can't understand why people can't move on. I did with all my losses ... each day I got a little better, it wasn't too long, I had to continue working, life had to go on and I got on with it. It sounds very cruel, sometimes I can't understand why other people can't do the same.'

This raises an important issue. If such a 'block' exists, an important first step is to acknowledge it. This worker went on to describe how she had to be very careful when working with the bereaved. This included not being judgemental and trying to understand when they are stuck and that with the best will in the world they cannot move on.

The difficulties that can occur when extrapolating from personal experience are also illustrated by a primary school teacher's reaction following the death of the mother of one of her pupils. At first the child didn't want to talk and there was no mention of her mother in her writing. She didn't appear to react at all. This reaction was different from what the teacher expected and she wasn't sure what to make of it. Her expectations were based on the reaction of her son, aged 8 years, when his grandmother died. He was devastated, distraught and angry. He blamed God and couldn't cope with the idea that his grandmother had gone into hospital and then died. It was not until several weeks after her mother's death that the pupil suddenly 'let it all out.' She sat on the teacher's knee crying for at least an hour and then fell asleep.

THE PROBLEM OF IDENTIFICATION

Vachon (1987) quotes several examples of the process of identification. One involved a young nurse who became very upset when a man died following neurosurgery. As she started talking to the chaplain, she realized that this patient reminded her of her husband, from whom she was divorced. She was still very upset regarding the divorce and the circumstances surrounding it. An unresolved loss in this nurse's life resulted in a very strong reaction following the death of a particular patient. Fortunately, she had help in recognizing the connection.

Sometimes the process of identification is more easily recognized. A cook in a small cottage hospital had quite regular contact with the patients. One of them looked very much like her dead father: not only did he have similar features but he also had beautiful hands like her father's. She clearly established excellent rapport with this patient. 'It was almost as if they'd given me back my dad for a short while, even if it was only visually. It was like thinking that every day I came to work, I'd be able to see dad in a way.' When she returned from 3 days leave, the bad news was broken to her that this patient had died. Her description of her reaction included 'It really upset me . . . I actually sat sobbing. But I don't know whether that was for the patient or because he reminded me so much of my dad . . . I thought about him quite a lot afterwards.'

Her response did not appear to be connected with unresolved feelings about her father's death. She only reported some guilt about not being with him when he died. Her experience highlights the importance of considering the effect of patient deaths on all staff. Nursing staff had been anxious about breaking the news of the patient's death; they didn't know how to tell her because they knew she would be upset. However, they were able to provide support by sitting her down, making her a cup of tea and having a nurse sit with her.

A general nurse working with older people, referring back to earlier in her career when she worked with children and younger adults, described her feelings. 'It was talking to the parents of seriously ill children. I felt for them, how they must be feeling. I was probably putting myself in their shoes. With seriously ill younger adults I felt extremely sorry for them, especially if they were leaving young children behind.'

At the time this nurse's own children were very young and she was probably identifying with the patients/families she was caring for. She used to think about them outside work and was noticeably quiet at home. At work she used to provide relief cover on different wards and sometimes staff used to comment on how quiet she was and ask what was the matter. Following this experience, she asked not to work on children's wards again and later made a conscious decision to work with older adults.

ACCUMULATED LOSS

Adams *et al.* (1991), in a study of 100 hospice caregivers, describe five characteristics of accumulated loss:

- **lack of closure**: lack of emotional processing because of insufficient opportunity to deal with death of patient and grief of family;
- **dying and death concerns**: thoughts or anxieties that are evoked – these could relate to personal or imagined scenarios of illness, disability and death;
- **ideals versus reality incongruity**: this is the discomfort or stress consequent upon the discrepancy between desired and actual clinical practice;
- **identification-distancing**: these are psychological strategies for separating self from pressures of clinical practice;
- **diminished boundaries**: when personal and care-giving commitments become blurred.

Cook and Oltjenbruns (1989) refer to the concept of accumulated loss but use different terminology. They use the term **bereavement overload**, which refers to the situation in which a griever must deal with several deaths in close succession and does not have the time to cope with the first death before another one comes along. Oltjenbruns (1987) has also coined the term **incremental grief**, which is the additive factor of grief due to multiple related losses. This is discussed in the context of primary and secondary loss. A primary loss would, for example, be the death of someone to whom one was close. If one's subsequent relationship with others who knew the deceased well becomes strained, then secondary loss can be experienced, i.e. grief over a deterioration in the pre-death relationship with these other people. So the grief resulting from a primary loss may trigger a secondary loss and then the grief associated with the secondary loss could lead to another loss – hence the term incremental grief. An example of incremental grief has been referred to above – ideals versus reality incongruity (Adams et al., 1991). The loss of a caregiver's idealized role expectations has also been referred to by Shanfield (1981). Medical and nursing training is focused on treating disease and saving lives, so in addition to grief following the death of a patient doctors and nurses are confronted with their limitations as professional caregivers. For some, patient death may be viewed as failure.

Another example of incremental grief following a patient's death is when the death has been difficult and involved conflict with other professionals. Saunders and Valente (1994) identify the task for nurses in this case as being the realigning of any disrupted relationships. Failure to do so may disrupt the work of the team. These authors also make the important point that the team as a whole, as well as individual members, may be susceptible to the cumulative effects of loss.

The problem for the professional caregiver in relation to accumulated loss is stated simply by Rando (1984): 'If accumulated grief is not worked through, the caregiver is every bit as vulnerable to all the malignant sequelae of unresolved grief as is any other individual who has suffered a loss but failed to complete his/her grief work.'

A hospice worker described to one of the authors how she recognized the effects of accumulated loss: 'I stop worrying and I wonder if I'm getting hardened . . . When I can't cry or I don't feel upset. Then I think, well, maybe it's time to move on . . . That mainly happens when it is one death after another.' She was then able to talk to her colleagues about how awful things were and that she couldn't cope with much more.

Awareness of the potential hazards of accumulated loss, not just patient deaths but also other losses, is an important first step that can lead on to working through the associated grief.

LOSS OF 'OUGHTS'

Loss is usually viewed as something that has happened i.e. an event. We talk, for example, of the death of a relative or loss of a job. However, there is another form of loss: the loss of something that ought to happen but probably never will. Part of the dictionary definition of 'ought' is: 'To express probability or expectation, to express a desire or wish on the part of the speaker' (Collins Concise English Dictionary, 1992).

Many loss of 'oughts' can also be described as non-event losses. One way in which the work of professional helpers can be affected by such losses is if one occurs in their personal lives. Larson (1993) quotes a nurse working in a maternity unit: 'I get so angry when mothers of healthy newborns use me as a baby sitter or refuse to care for their own baby when I have been trying desperately to conceive a child of my own.'

Stewart and Dent (1994) point out that there is significant grief following miscarriage even though there is no tangible loss. The 'ought' loss is that the fetus should have developed into a healthy baby. A generic social worker interviewed by one of the authors had experienced several miscarriages and she managed to successfully avoid work involving children. She always had an excuse such as already having a large caseload.

It is possible that these two workers still have unresolved grief issues around in relation to their loss of 'oughts.' This makes it difficult to work with clients who have got what they, the carers, ought to have.

Another way that such losses can affect professional carers is through identifying with loss of 'oughts' in clients. Shanfield (1981) mentions a medical student who cried when he learned that a young man with schizophrenia had a poor prognosis. He was identifying with the young man's future loss of career, upward mobility and success. A hospice worker who had cared for teenagers with leukaemia commented: 'I think of where I was at their time of life and I look at all the opportunities that they may miss.' A nurse with experience of caring for the terminally ill commented: 'Patients say to you, "I thought I'd see my grandchildren." You have empathy with that patient because **you** want to see **your** grandchildren.'

It is the view of the authors that grief associated with loss of 'oughts' is an important area that is not usually considered because people do not normally think about loss in this way.

In this chapter we have explored the grief that professional helpers can experience at work and some of the factors that can influence this. We have also considered the positive impact of loss experiences and how awareness of the more negative aspects can be helpful. In particular we have highlighted the importance of the interaction between personal and professional aspects of loss.

The reader may find it helpful to consider some of the following questions, which aim to raise awareness of the interplay between personal and professional issues and how this might affect work with people experiencing loss.

Self-awareness exercise – Personal/professional issues in working with loss

- How has my work with people experiencing loss affected my attitude to life? Can I use this positively in my work?
- Do any of the following words or phrases describe my reactions to people I have cared for:
  - over-reacting, e.g. very upset or exceptionally nice/making an extra effort;
  - rejecting or avoiding;
  - envious;
  - possessive;
  - the worst person I have looked after;
  - the best person I have looked after?

If so, could there be a connection with my own losses, or past or present relationships in my life?

- Which clients/patients remind me of people I've known in a positive way?
- Which clients/patients remind me of people I've known in a negative way?
- How is the way I relate to these clients/patients affected?
- Do some clients/patients remind me of a significant person in my life who has died? If so, does this affect how I relate to them?
- Do I ever judge how my clients/patients will feel or react on the basis of my personal experience of loss? If so, is this helpful or not?
- Are there losses in my own life that I may not have properly dealt with? If so, could this be affecting my work?
- Are there things that ought to have happened in my life that could be affecting my work?
- Which clients/patients or families am I more likely to identify with?
- What loss of 'oughts' in clients/patients or families am I more likely to identify with?
- When I experience an accumulation of losses in a short period of time, how does this affect me and how do I deal with it emotionally?

Feared loss – can it affect our work?

5

I get upset at the thought of something happening to my kids. I'd be at risk if my kids were to die. I ask myself how I'd cope if my husband were to die – that's in part why I went back to work, to be an independent, self-contained person, not just his wife. I think I could cope if he were to die but my kids are a different story.

Volunteer co-ordinator quoted in Vachon, 1987

To be of most service to others, a person must first face personal needs and doubts.

Dass and Gorman, 1985

It's just the thought of never seeing things again, never being able to see my children's faces change as they grow up or never seeing grandchildren if I had any. The things that I would lose out on personally. I'd rather lose a leg or an arm than lose the capability of doing that.

General nurse

It does not seem to be culturally acceptable to think of the future in any negative way. We are encouraged to look on the bright side or to think positive. Thinking about the possibility of adverse events is usually delayed, as encapsulated in the saying, 'I'll cross that bridge when I come to it.' Problems are dealt with only when they arise.

Hand in hand with this emphasis on being positive is a common suspicion that if one talks about something bad it will happen or increase the chance that it might happen. In workshops run by the authors, the issue of wills often arises and often many participants have not made a will. Some are actively discouraged from doing so by their partners. Talking about matters following one's death is viewed as tempting fate.

It is difficult for all concerned to cope with a major loss. This is illustrated by some of the unhelpful responses made at such times. Those mentioned by Lendrum and Syme (1992) include:

- 'Every cloud has a silver lining.'
- 'There's light at the end of the tunnel.'
- 'Of course you'll find someone else.'
- 'You'll get over it.'

Welch *et al.* (1991) refer to this kind of comment as cliché statements. Two examples from their list are:

- 'It was for the best.'
- 'You must be strong for your children.'

Shapiro (1988) mentions the kinds of comment that are made to people who have fertility problems or who lose a pregnancy, for instance:

- 'It's important not to give up.'
- 'You can try again.'

Grollman (1990) quotes an example of an unhelpful comment made to a child following the death of a pet dog: 'Why are you crying so hard? It's only a dog. It's not as if something happened to your parents. We can always buy another pet.'

If we are not very good at talking about or listening to the pain of loss when it happens, how can we possibly think about such eventualities in advance? Isn't it just being unnecessarily morbid? What is the point of distressing ourselves by thinking about such things? Deits (1992) suggests that it is possible to prepare for loss: 'Getting in touch with your feelings about the possibility of such events is a way of beginning to prepare for losses that are unavoidable'.

Feared loss can be defined as any potential loss that causes us to feel uneasy, anxious or low in mood when we think about it. One of the authors has quite a lot of videotapes of his children playing, for instance in school concerts and various musical events. The thought of these tapes being stolen in a burglary causes some uneasiness because they are irreplaceable. This is an example of the 'lower end' of feared loss. At the other extreme, the thought of the death of a loved one could cause very high levels of distress.

The specific feared loss of one's own death is discussed in Chapter 6. However, there are parallels between considering mortality and feared loss in general. Saunders and Valente (1994) point out that existentialists suggest that most people survive day-to-day life by ignoring the reality that they might die at any moment. A death can shake one's illusion of security. To face feared loss is to be confronted with the fact that nothing is permanent. Referring back to the light bulb analogy in Chapter 4, the filament could blow at any moment. A loved one could die at any time. The possibility of such loss was brought home to one of the authors while writing this chapter. On Saturday 15 June 1996 a bomb exploded in the centre of Manchester, UK and a few Saturdays prior to this he had been fairly close to where the explosion took place at the same time of day with two members of his family. Deits (1992) points out that loss is an inescapable part of being alive and makes some stark points, including the fact that every marriage ends in one of two ways: death or divorce, every career has an end and the ageing process is inevitable.

In this chapter we will discuss how considering and being aware of feared loss can assist a professional helper in working more effectively. Some of the potential hazards of thinking about feared loss will also be addressed.

THE RELATIONSHIP BETWEEN PERCEIVED LEVEL OF VALUE AND FEARED LOSS

Imagine that you had a car that was unreliable and becoming expensive to keep on the road. Assuming you could replace the car, you would probably have a low fear of it being stolen. You might even wish that it would be stolen, so you could claim the insurance money. This is an example of how low perceived value is often associated with low feared loss (quadrant A in Figure 5.1).

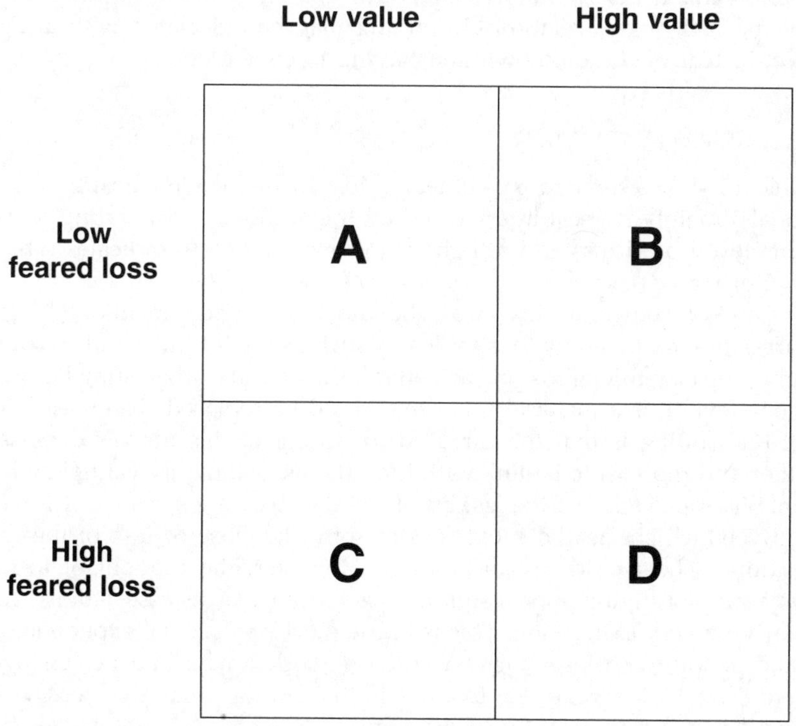

	Low value	High value
Low feared loss	A	B
High feared loss	C	D

Figure 5.1   The loss and value window.

At the other extreme, high value is usually associated with high feared loss. Two of the quotes at the beginning of this chapter, relating to the prospect of one's children dying and losing one's sight, illustrate this. In relation to the work of a helping professional, this relationship (quadrant D in Figure 5.1) is probably the most important. Quadrant B, i.e. high value and low feared loss, suggests that something may have 'gone wrong'. For example, a once dedicated helping professional may be feeling undervalued and on the verge of becoming burnt out. He/she may cease to treat clients as individuals, lose previous job satisfaction and no longer care about continuing to do the job. The perceived value of the work may still be high but the fear of losing one's position has become low because of a strong build-up of negative factors.

Quadrant C is perhaps the most difficult to interpret. Low value may be associated with high feared loss in the context of a lot of other losses. A further loss, however minor, could be the straw that might break the camel's back. Another possibility is that something may have low value when compared with other potential losses but be associated with high feared loss because of personal significance. An example of this might be a memento that links one to somebody who has died. It is also possible that a stormy, ambivalent relationship may not be highly valued but the fear of this relationship ending may be associated with a high level of fear of the unknown and having to cope alone.

RATINGS OF FEARED LOSS

Table 5.1 shows some ratings of feared loss made by a few health professionals (mainly nurses) interviewed by the authors. A low rating represents low feared loss and a high rating (maximum 10) indicates a high level of feared loss.

Death of someone close was the most frequently mentioned high feared loss, followed by 'health' losses such as loss of independence and sight. The example of loss of car with a rating of 10 is interesting because at one level it is a material thing that could be replaced. The reason for the high rating is that the car used to belong to this nurse's deceased father and represented a link with him. It was also highly valued by her son. She reported, 'It's the last bit of my dad we've got really.' If forced to say which she feared most, loss of someone close or loss of the car, no doubt she would say the former. However, the thought of losing something of high personal significance (because of its associations) can clearly be very distressing. This is borne out by the actual experience of some people who lose rings. A support worker who had her engagement ring stolen reported to one of the authors that this was very distressing (a rating of 9 on a 10-point scale where 0 = not distressing at all and 10 = extremely distressing). Another worker who had her

Table 5.1   Some feared loss ratings of health professionals

Feared loss	Rating
Death of people close to	
Children	10
Husband	10
Grandchildren	10
Close friends	10, 9
Boyfriend	10
Parent	10, 8, 6
Siblings	7
Health loss	
Sight	10
Independence/mobility	10, 9
Sanity (e.g. from dementia)	10
From ageing process	9
Limb	6
Illness of children	6
Psychological/social loss	
Loss of awareness of others' needs (becoming hardened)	10
Loss of motivation to pursue knowledge and learning	10
Loss of the familiar	8
Divorce	6
Social status/standards	4
Spiritual loss	
Loss of appreciation for the beauty and creation in the world	10
Loss of job/income	
My job	10, 8, 6
Husband's job	10
Income	4
Loss of possessions	
Car that belonged to deceased father	10
House burglary	6
Loss of pet	
Dog	6

wedding ring and her engagement ring stolen in a burglary rated this
as fairly distressing (about 6 on the scale). The individual variation and
highly personal nature of such losses is illustrated by a nurse who lost
her wedding ring; she described it as a little loss.

Fear of loss of job was mentioned a few times. The degree of this
depended upon personal circumstances: for instance, the rating of 10
was from somebody who had no other source of income. The high
rating for loss of husband's job was because he was seen as the main
breadwinner.

Many of the psychological losses were mentioned by a social worker. The high ratings seem to relate to fear of becoming burnt out. She also mentioned the spiritual fear of not being able to appreciate the world around her.

These kinds of feared loss are similar to those raised in workshops run by the authors. The most feared losses are usually close family members and poor physical or mental health in oneself or family members. Others include loss of wider relationships such as friends and extended family and more personal things like a sense of purpose and hope. Over the course of several workshops, participants have also shown the kind of variation in feared loss discussed above. For example, for loss of job, 16 participants gave a rating from 8–10, 17 a rating from 5–7 and seven a rating from 0–4. Similar wide variability has been shown for loss of pets, home, car and possessions such as jewellery. Even though feared loss in relation to health is usually high, some people give lower ratings. Examples of the latter are a finger or toe, teeth, loss of energy, mobility, memory and senses such as sight and hearing.

FEARED LOSS, INVOLVEMENT AND DEPENDENCY

The high feared loss in relation to significant others referred to above is likely to be even more extreme if there is a high level of involvement with and dependency on these other persons. Parkes (1996) alludes to the possible effects of such involvement: 'the greater the area occupied by A in the life-space of B, the greater the disruption that will result from A's departure'. If the dependency on a significant other takes the form of a strong, insecure attachment (e.g. with elements of 'clinging' and anxiety) the thought of losing this person may evoke very high feared loss.

FEARED LOSS AND AGE

The nature of feared loss is likely to vary according to the stage of the life cycle we are at. Someone in their twenties or thirties may be concerned, for example, about career development, possible loss of job and family security. An older retired person may be more concerned about being sufficiently healthy to pursue interests or about possible loss of independence if health deteriorates, and also about grandchildren as well as children. An illustration of how priorities may be different is an older man, seen by one of the authors, who had suffered a stroke. He reported that what he missed most was playing physical games with his grandchildren.

Given the previous discussion about the relationship between value and feared loss, changes in feared loss with age may be partly accounted for by changes in what is valued as we get older, as well as life events.

In some respects feared loss may be reduced with older age; for example, we may not have to worry so much about maintaining a stable reputation. A poem by Joseph (1996) is a humorous illustration of this: it describes what a woman will do when she gets old – wear purple with a red hat that doesn't suit her and learn to spit and generally make up for the sobriety of her youth. Maggie Kuhn, leader of the Gray Panther movement in America, also explained when speaking in the United Kingdom in 1985 (Central Independent Television, 1985) why she thought older people were better placed to change things in society: 'We have nothing to lose, nothing. We've already lost our jobs through mandatory retirement, many of us have lost loved ones, spouses, children even and place in society. We have nothing to lose, we can take the risks ... We're free, we can speak our minds.'

One implication is that professional helpers should not assume that their feared losses are the same as their clients', especially if the clients are much older or younger.

HOW CAN FEARED LOSS AFFECT US?

A HEIGHTENED SENSE OF WHAT IS VALUED

Consider the situation of a single parent who ponders the possibility that his/her child might die first. What thoughts or feelings might be going through this parent's mind?

Some insight into this can be gained from the actual experience of a single parent whose child died, aged 22 years, in an automobile accident. Gillis (1993) talks of the loss of a companion and helpmate and the end of family life. One day she was parenting and the next, nothing. She would never again hear those words 'Hi, Mom'. She also describes some of the other associated losses:

> Gone are the graduations, birthday parties, proms and the dream of my child's wedding. The thought of Christmas in my home ... without this precious person, is unbearable ... I will never become a grandparent, never see my family grow through my daughter and her family ... Never again in social situations will I be able to say, 'This is my daughter Lorena' and know the love and pride I felt in having her.

This parent also observes that before her daughter's death she did not realize how much the question, 'How many children do you have?' was part of her life. This seems to relate to the issue of taking people/ situations for granted. Lagrande (1988) quotes a young woman whose mother and brother died: 'If you love someone, let them know it now. They might not be here tomorrow.' A hospice worker involved in the care of a young man with cancer had a son of a similar age. When thinking about this young man's mother she thought, 'There but for the grace of God go I.' She reported: 'I would go home and look at my son and I'd say, "Oh give me a cuddle," and he'd say, "Oh mum, what for?" I'd say, "Just give me a cuddle."'

These observations illustrate one advantage of considering feared loss; it highlights those important aspects of life that are highly valued and precious to us and makes it less likely that we will take them for granted. Part of this awareness comes from considering all the manifestations of a loss as illustrated in the first example above. An experienced general nurse took part in a workshop exercise in which she had to 'give up' important people and things in her life. This created a horrible feeling in her and she was thankful it wasn't real. However, she described the personal benefits: 'It made me prioritize my life in a way. I was so glad that I still have my family, my sight and my mobility. I am more affectionate towards my husband and I want him to know that I appreciate he is here. It really made me think and appreciate more.'

This illustrates an important point made by Deits (1992) – that the greatest benefit of preparing for loss is probably not what it does for life after loss, but what it does for life before loss.

UNHELPFUL EFFECT ON BEHAVIOUR

Feared loss is not just a vague notion that may unsettle us a little if we think about it. It can also affect behaviour. An example of this is the fear of losing a child in a parent with a history of infertility. Shapiro (1988) quotes a parent who was very overprotective and always aware of dangers or risks. This parent, for example, used to check the child two or three times a night, used a car seat for an extra year and never let the child ride in cars driven by other parents. The most revealing part of the parent's statement is: 'Since, deep down, I was terrified of losing her, I spent a lot of energy anticipating possible threats and protecting her against them.'

This kind of overprotection may make a child unnecessarily wary and insecure. Fear of losing a much loved child may also result in parents wanting to conceive or adopt another child as soon as possible. This 'future child' may be seen as a replacement for the possible loss that they dread. Vachon (1987) mentions a funeral director, who reported that if he married he would not just have one child but would probably have up to three or four. From his work he was aware that children can die. It could be argued that this kind of fear alone is not a sound basis on which to base family planning.

A social worker admitted to not being very good with elderly people. 'I see myself there and I'm afraid of the ageing process. I wouldn't want to be dependent upon others.' She was sometimes impatient and not very tolerant when working with older people and their carers.

In a later section we will consider how feared loss can lead to avoidance of working with certain client groups and point out that this need not necessarily be unhelpful.

HELPFUL EFFECT ON BEHAVIOUR

Feared loss can be put to good use. It can help to constructively empathize with clients. The experienced general nurse mentioned earlier in the section 'A heightened sense of what is valued' also described the professional benefits of considering feared loss. She works on a long-stay ward for physically frail older men.

> It made me really think what it must be like for people who have lost all these things. One of my patients can get very awkward if you can't understand him. You ask him to write it down and he writes a swear word. I used to get very uptight. Now I see him in a different light, I can understand why he reacts in this way. I ignore the swear words and have more patience in trying to find out what he wants.

So awareness of one's feared losses can provide motivation to give good quality care. The following examples illustrate this in relation to fear of loss of independence. A hospice social worker reported: 'With some illnesses I would be dependent upon others. I would be a burden to people and I would hate it if perhaps my mental faculties were there but physically I couldn't even wipe a tear from my eye or blow my own nose. I would prefer to be dead. That terrifies me in some ways.'

Because this was an important issue for her, she felt it was important that patients should keep as much control over their own lives as possible and this influenced her practice. This worker specifically mentioned fear of developing Alzheimer's disease, not only because of becoming dependent on others but also because of failing mental faculties. This fear appeared to make her more determined when earlier in her career she worked with patients with Alzheimer's disease and their carers: 'I suppose because I felt so strongly about it ... not anger, but passion ... more passion to get where I wanted to go for that family, or that patient, I think would overcome any of my own sort of fears. But I suppose it could be fear in me that drove me to that passion.'

A hospice nurse wondered how she would accept losing her independence. This was at the forefront of her mind after her mother suffered a slight stroke. She contemplated whether she would like to be dependent on her own children. She summed up her fear: 'I should hate to be totally dependent on another person, for example, having a stroke, losing my speech. That would worry me. I must admit, in all honesty, that of the things that have bothered me recently, that's been one of them.'

The effect on this nurse was to make her more sensitive and aware of the feelings of patients and their families. She described how this translated into practice: 'It makes me more aware of patients' need to protect their dignity and that I shouldn't talk over them and down to them. With families, that we shouldn't take over, but give them space to say, "We can't cope" or "We need more help"'.

THE CLIENTS WE PREFER NOT TO WORK WITH

Several nurses have reported to the authors how difficult experiences of working with children have led to them avoiding this area of work. An example was mentioned in Chapter 4. It is also possible that fear of loss may lead to avoidance of nursing children. This is illustrated by a general nurse who feared personal involvement and identifying with parents both in her personal and professional life:

My godson was born 13 weeks premature but I would not go and see him because I didn't want to pick him up and hold him unless I knew that he was going to survive. I detached myself from him because I didn't want to become personally involved. I think the danger of becoming very personally involved is that you feel the loss about as much as the parents do. You think about how you would feel if it was your child who was ill. It was because of this that I chose not to work with children.

A critical element in such fear seems to be the factors in one's personal life that make identification more likely. For helpers with children, the ages of their offspring are clearly important. Also, an older nurse reported to one of the authors that she felt she wouldn't be very good working with children because she had two young grandchildren.

Pines (1982) reported how fear of a baby dying while having an operation can affect work and quotes the example of an anaesthetist who had a 'soft spot' for babies and had great difficulty anaesthetizing them in the operating room. She had nightmares in which she was haunted by dead babies with dilated pupils for some weeks after such operations. The hospital would not be flexible and allow her not to work with babies and this was a major factor in her having to take a year off work.

As Buckman (1996a) has pointed out, the word 'cancer' can cause mental paralysis and terror and this is partly the result of lack of knowledge and understanding. Cancer is actually a group of 200 diseases. Some skin cancers are 99% curable and some cancers, e.g. advanced cancer of the pancreas, will lead to death in months. Then there are a range of cancers in between these extremes. Approximately half of all cancers will be cured by an initial operation. Despite these observations, which support the statement that the disease is not a single entity with one uniformly bad prognosis, the reader will recall from Chapter 4 that Lerea and LiMauro (1982) found that cancer was the diagnosis that elicited grief most often for nurses. A general nurse reported to one of the authors that she didn't know whether she could nurse cancer patients. This reluctance, although partly connected with experience of cancer in her family, also appeared to be related to fear of the disease.

All professional helpers have strengths and weaknesses and awareness of our feared losses may help to make decisions about which clients we can work with most effectively. It may also be useful to be aware that fear of a particular area of work may be based on misunderstandings, as in the case of oncology mentioned above.

DIFFICULT PERSONAL ISSUES CAN BE EVOKED

Although the authors are convinced of the potential benefits of considering feared loss, there are risks involved. A staff nurse was reluctant to take part in a feared loss exercise in which she might have to consider the possibility of people close to her dying, particularly her father, to whom she was very close. In a later discussion, one of her colleagues pointed out that 'this is life' and these things do happen, quoting the example of someone she knew, whose family had been 'wiped out' in a car accident. Some people are not persuaded by such arguments and the process of thinking about possible future losses can evoke difficult issues and even be traumatic.

A nurse who was making some feared loss ratings at home reported that it was terrible and really got to her. It made her feel depressed, she kept putting it off and it took her a long time to complete. She had experienced several losses and the thought of anything happening to her children, for instance, caused a high level of anxiety. When asked to imagine the death of a significant person with no-one else close to her to confide in, this nurse felt she could be suicidal. Another nurse, asked the same question, used words like 'desperate' to describe how she thought she would feel.

A nurse who took part in the feared loss exercise referred to earlier, in which one has to give up/lose important people or things in one's life, had a very negative reaction. She had written down on cards the names of a few significant people in her life and chose one at random to 'lose.' This turned out to be her daughter and she thought 'Oh no!' and put the card back. She had always been very fond of children and had found it too difficult to care for dying children in a professional role. Hence the exercise touched a sensitive area for her. She also reported some difficulty in grieving for her father, who had died 8 years previously: she bottled up her feelings and couldn't talk about him for a long time. She also still had some guilt feelings related to his death. Anticipating the possibility of the death of other significant people could have reawakened these difficulties related to the death of her father. Other factors that could have made considering future loss difficult included a tendency to put a brave face on and to put others' needs before her own. Her family did not show their feelings much and she could never discuss death with her husband, who could not be persuaded to make a will. It is important to note, however, that even though this nurse had a negative reaction to considering feared loss, she did admit that it made her more aware of what it would be like to lose, for instance, one of her children.

When asking staff to engage in feared loss exercises it is important to consider making backup support available so there is an opportunity to discuss difficult issues that may be evoked. There is a risk that, without careful introduction and debriefing, staff may be left with feelings of, for instance, shock, sadness and guilt that have not been emotionally processed, particularly if they continue to have feelings of anger directed at the person who 'put them through it'.

In this chapter we have discussed the nature of feared loss and its relationship to perceived level of value, involvement/dependency and age. We have highlighted some of the benefits of considering feared loss, including how it can increase empathy with clients and have a direct positive effect on practice. Some problems have also been explored – how it can affect ability to work with particular client groups and raise difficult personal issues. It is hoped that raising awareness of the issue of feared loss will assist the reader in putting it to constructive use.

Some feared loss trigger questions are presented below and it is recommended that the reader considers them together with a colleague, so there is opportunity for mutual exploration and support.

Some feared loss questions to consider

- Which of my senses would I least like to lose? Why?
- How would I react if I were to lose my mobility and independence?
- Of the significant people in my life, whose death would be the most difficult to cope with? Why?
- Overall, what do I value most highly in my life? Do I ever take this for granted?
- Is considering feared loss very painful for me? If so, what could be the reasons for this?
- Do I have any feared losses that make it difficult to work with particular client groups?

- What is the discrepancy between my age and the average age of my clients? Are my feared losses likely to be similar to those of my clients or their relatives?
- How can awareness of my feared losses increase my empathy with clients? How can I translate this into more effective practice?

Thinking about our own death

6

The weariest and most loathed worldly life
That age, ache, penury and imprisonment
Can lay on nature, is a paradise
To what we fear of death.

William Shakespeare: Measure for Measure Act III Scene 1

The meanings we assign to death help shape our pastoral response to loss,
to dying and bereavement.

Griffin, 1990

I've never had a big operation like this before and it's the fear of not
waking up from the anaesthetic . . . It's the thought of going in there and
that's it and not knowing what's on the other side and of all the things
that I won't have said before I go.

General nurse

According to Littlewood (1992) death has been 'conjured away' from our culture. It is something we don't normally talk about, so why is it important that helping professionals should consider their own death? The main reason is that if we have unspoken fears and anxieties about death, this will act as a barrier and prevent us from truly getting alongside dying people. It may even lead to avoiding the dying. In this chapter we consider the importance of personal beliefs and anxieties, as well as various ways of thinking about death, including philosophical and theological positions.

The work of Feifel and colleagues in the 1960s (Feifel, 1965; Feifel *et al.*, 1967) suggested that doctors had a greater fear of death than other groups. From this it was thought that they might have chosen to work in the medical field in an attempt to achieve mastery over illness and thereby deal with their fear of death. However, in reviewing later studies Neimeyer and Van Brunt (1995) concluded that medical professionals are not significantly more apprehensive about death and dying than other groups. If physicians do maintain a view of themselves as omnipotent healers as a way of mitigating their fear of death, then Lev (1989) suggests that this may interfere with their self-awareness and ability to give care. We will now review some studies which relate fear of death in doctors and nurses more specifically to various aspects of care.

CAN FEARS ABOUT DEATH AFFECT CARE?

Wilkinson (1991) carried out a study with 54 nurses caring for cancer patients. This included consideration of blocking verbal behaviours such as ignoring, changing the topic of conversation and giving inappropriate advice. One of the factors that influenced the use of these blocking verbal behaviours was the nurse's fear about her own death, as measured by a fear of death scale (Collett and Lester, 1969). Those who had most fear of dying blocked patients more frequently. They protected themselves from being reminded of death and dying by not allowing themselves to be subjected to patients' emotions and distress.

In another study with 312 nurses (qualified and assistants) Hare and Pratt (1989) considered the relationship between fear of death and comfort level in working with dying patients. The latter was assessed by ratings of questions such as, 'How comfortable are you with sitting down for at least 10 minutes with such a patient when you believe he or she would like to talk about his or her feelings?' Three aspects of fear of death were assessed: fear of the dying process, fear of premature death and fear for significant others. The last two of these were significantly negatively correlated with nurses' level of comfort in caring for dying patients. So the greater the fear of death, the lower the comfort level.

Schulz and Aderman (1979) asked 24 hospital physicians to complete a death anxiety scale (developed by Sarnoff and Corwin, 1959) over the telephone. Following investigation of hospital records, they found that patients of physicians with high death anxiety were in hospital an average of 5 days longer before dying than patients treated by physicians with medium and low death anxiety. There were no significant differences in other measures such as time in hospital for other patients. The implication is that physicians with high death anxiety may do everything in their power to save patients, as a way of denying the impending death.

In a further study of doctors Barroso et al. (1992) carried out a questionnaire study of 153 Spanish physicians. Those who agreed or strongly agreed with the statement 'Dying patients should never be made aware that they are dying' had a greater fear of dying (as measured by statements such as 'I am very worried about suffering a slow painful death' and 'I would like to be unconscious during my death'). These authors suggest that although physicians cannot be immune to cultural influences, they should reflect critically on their personal attitudes and how these affect their professional decisions.

Similar recommendations for physicians to consider personal factors affecting their decision making processes were made by Eggerman and Dustin (1985) following their study of 103 medical students, eight physician assistants and 15 family physicians. They found, for example, that physicians who were less likely to identify their own death with the death of a terminally ill patient were more likely to consider an increased number of support variables before making a decision of whether to tell the patient that he or she was terminally ill. Support variables included the support of family and friends and depth of religious faith.

These studies of nurses and doctors suggest that professional helpers' fears about their own deaths can affect the physical and emotional care they provide, how they feel and decisions about informing patients of their diagnosis and prognosis. This points to the potential value of considering personal issues to do with death, which may reduce underlying fears.

WHAT DO PROFESSIONAL HELPERS THINK ABOUT DEATH?

In workshops we ask people to consider various issues relating to their own death. One question is: 'What would you do with your life if you knew that in 6 months you would die?' Welch *et al.* (1991) pose various alternative responses to this kind of question, including putting things in order, indulging oneself and being concerned with the needs of one's family. We have found the latter two responses to be quite common. People want to give up work, go on holiday (e.g. a cruise) and generally do things they have always wanted to do. Alternatively, they want to support family members and generally help them to prepare for life after their death. An example of the latter was given by one of the nurses we interviewed, who would want her significant others to be left as intact as possible: 'If I had 6 months to live, I would want to make sure that everybody who was important to me knew how I felt about them and that we would support each other. I would not want to leave them blown apart and distraught to bits. That would be more important to me than an exotic holiday.'

For this nurse specific examples included telling her husband that she wouldn't mind if he got married again but would he please leave it a decent time. Also, discussing everyday practical matters such as making sure that their daughter went to school in her school uniform and that her hair was brushed.

Another question is: 'Which three people would you want at your death bed?' Again there is variability in the responses. Some would want close family members, others would prefer friends. The latter is illustrated in the following comments: 'I couldn't cope with the thought of my son and his hurt at my bedside'; 'I don't want my husband there weeping and wailing all over the place'. For some, three people is not enough; they want all close family members or all close friends present.

Two people we interviewed were particularly concerned about issues of dependency and loss of control and made comments such as: 'I wouldn't like to be bedfast and not be aware and not be in control. That's what bothers me, not being in control and just being left to linger.' In a situation of being highly dependent on others and feeling a burden one of these interviewees felt she would be terrified and probably prefer to be dead. Some professionals find it too difficult to address issues relating to their own death and will find that they cannot answer the kinds of question mentioned above. They may feel it would be tempting fate.

These insights may help in understanding what dying people may be experiencing or are concerned about. Also, our concerns about dying may not be the same as people who are actually dying. Sometimes people hang on to normality as an anchor point (Chapter 1). Many would probably want close family members at their death bed but, as illustrated above, not everybody would necessarily want this. Sometimes our own anxieties may make it difficult to care for some people, as in the example of fear of dependency and loss of control mentioned above. The most important first step is to go through the process of addressing our own thoughts and feelings about death, even if this leads to a realization that we cannot properly address them. The resulting awareness will make us more sensitive as to how our concerns may affect the care we provide.

WORDS ASSOCIATED WITH DEATH

Before reading this section the reader may wish to write down three words that he or she associates with death, so that a comparison can be made with the thoughts of other professionals. Stewart and Dent (1994) have found in workshops with professionals that many are frightened of pain, of being isolated, of being dependent and of losing control. Also, for some death was the end, for others it was a new beginning. Many were uncertain and for most dying was more frightening than death itself. Welch et al. (1991) mention common fears of death and dying, including what happens after death (e.g. nothingness, no life after death), fear of the process of dying (e.g. pain and indignity) and loss of life in general (e.g. loss of control, separation from loved ones).

In our workshops with various professionals (a high proportion of whom were nurses) we have asked participants to note down three words that reflect how they feel about death in general. Table 6.1 represents a categorization of these words and it will be noted that most of the

Table 6.1 Categorization of words associated with death among health professionals

Fear	Other strong negative feelings	Other troublesome feelings	Loss	Philosophy – the end	Uncertainty	Philosophical attitude	Positive aspects	Spiritual/religious
Fear (13)	Anger (3)	Sad (11)	Loss (8)	Final (9)	Timing/when? (2)	Inevitable (10)	Peace (8)	Hope (3)
Apprehensive (4)	Cheated	Loneliness (5)	Loss of control	Ending (2)	What die of?	Unknown (7)	Relief (6)	Curiosity (3)
Scared (3)	Waste	Pain (4)	Parting	Emptiness (2)	Ambiguous	Part of life (2)	Release (3)	Intrigue
Anxious (2)	Unacceptable	Sorrow (3)	Separation	Non-existent (2)	Ambivalent	Unavoidable	Pain-free (2)	Deep
Frightened	Abandonment	Disbelief	Loss of contact	Permanent		Compulsory	Escape	Optimism
Terrified	Premature	Denial		Fading away		Equality	Comfort	Penultimate
Afraid	Devastating	Helplessness		End of life		Natural	Calm	Heaven
Worrying	Horrible	Guilt		Forever (dead)		Change	Dignity	Better life
	Horrendous	Isolated				Indiscriminate	A blessing	Rewarding
	Adversarial	Depressing				Eventful	Rest	A new beginning
	Invader	Burden				Already decided (fate)	Love	Another journey
		Suffering				Bargaining	Resolving conflict	Moving on
		Cold					Relatives closer	
		Darkness					Acceptance	Excitement

NB. Figures in parentheses indicate the number of times the word was mentioned across various workshops (no parentheses indicate word was mentioned once).

observations of Stewart and Dent (1994) and the kinds of fear mentioned by Welch *et al.* (1991) are included in this table.

The most commonly mentioned psychological concerns were:

- fear and associated feelings such as apprehension, anxiety and being scared;
- troublesome feelings of sadness, loneliness, pain and sorrow;
- loss such as loss of contact and parting.

Another less frequently mentioned psychological category was that of strong negative feelings other than fear. The most negative of these are perhaps feelings like devastation, horror and anger.

Under the philosophical headings, the most frequently mentioned themes were:

- Death is the end, i.e. it is final.
- It is inevitable.
- It is an unknown quantity.

Uncertainty about death was a less frequently mentioned theme and comments on positive aspects were more common. The latter consisted mainly of peace and the notion of relief or escape from suffering. Spiritual and religious aspects were mentioned less frequently than some of the other categories but covered a range of issues, including hope, curiosity and moving on to something new or something better.

PHILOSOPHICAL AND RELIGIOUS PERSPECTIVES ON DEATH

Some of the themes mentioned above illustrate the uncertainty in late twentieth century Western thinking regarding the meaning of death. It is seen as inevitable and final but what it means is uncertain.

Death is not something that human beings find easy to come to terms with. It presents us with a dilemma. Life as we now experience it would not be possible without death. We could probably not have the degree of joy associated with birth without the sadness of death. The sense of our own mortality can be one of the driving forces in our lives that give us a sense of ambition and desire for fulfilment. Yet most of us recoil at the prospect of our own death, seeing it as something entirely unnatural. Barroso *et al.* (1992), in the study of 153 randomly chosen doctors mentioned earlier, found that there was a greater aversion to death in urban environments than in rural ones. This may have a bearing on a society that is increasingly urban in nature. Yet, as Griffin (1990) writes, 'Without death we could not be human, but death takes from us all that is recognizably human.'

The failure to make sense of the meaning of death is often accompanied by no clear view as to the meaning of life either. This malaise in thinking about man's purpose is reflected in a search for personal meaning. This ranges, for example, from science to astrology, and from new age thinking to traditional religious thinking.

For some, death is something that happens to other people and it may never be considered in a personal sense. Intellectual assent can be given to the notion of the inevitability of our own death but the timing of it may be projected many years into the future. It is 'something we don't need to think about yet'. Talking about our own death or making any sort of plan for it is considered morbid and not to be encouraged. Such people 'do not see' a funeral procession as it passes them or treat the cortege as if it were just another series of cars. This was illustrated for one of the authors when, before a funeral, cones had been placed on the road outside the church to warn motorists that funeral cars would need to stop there. Ten minutes before the service a sales representative parked in the coned-off area. When reminded that the space was needed, he refused to move until the funeral procession was almost upon him.

For others death has no meaning, just as life has no meaning, unless we choose to give meaning to it. This is the view propagated by the existentialist philosophers, notably Kierkegaard, Heidegger and Sartre. As Cook (1988) writes, 'The existentialist believes that there is no meaning in any one thing, or in everything put together. The world is absurd and pointless. To be human is to choose in the light of the absurdity of the world.' Among the popular meanings given to human existence is the idea that death has meaning if life itself has had meaning. Another sees life as potentially going on for ever with each generation helping to improve the lot of the one following and of life being invested in the lives of our children. Many of us share at least an element of this way of thinking and this contributes to the great difficulty we have when one of our own children dies before we do. A further similar view on human existence also shares some Hindu and Buddhist thinking. It is a belief that life is like a relay baton passed on from one generation to the next. For these people, though, it is not the investment in ideas or discoveries that is primary but the passing on of genes. 'I live on after I die because some of my genes are carried in my children.' These philosophies are not always expressed very clearly but can be seen in the nature of some remarks that people make. For instance, one of the authors remembers a man at a funeral saying, 'It's strange, isn't it, how life goes on. George died on Tuesday and his grandchild was born on the Thursday.'

For Hindus and Buddhists life and death are but elements in the cycle of existence. How we live affects how we will be reborn into the cycle of life. Death therefore becomes no more than a transition from one life to another. Hinduism and Buddhism differ from each other in this respect in that for Hindus the goal is absorption into the deity while for Buddhists it is the reaching of the state of Nirvana or oneness with the universe. For Jews, Christians and Moslems death is the gateway either to eternal life or to judgement.

Hinton (1972) writes, 'Most societies . . . have comforting beliefs that temporal life on earth is but one aspect of total human existence' and 'Many take comfort from a belief in eventual rebirth after death, with the promise that death only interrupts life and that there will be a return to the wanted familiar world.' Griffin (1990) comments that in all religions the shared assumptions about death belief can no longer be taken for granted. He says, 'There is no one integrated set of beliefs to which all, or most, are likely to hold.'

Clearly there are a wide range of philosophical and religious perspectives on death and we have only mentioned some in this section. Our own views will not only affect the way we perceive our own death but also the way we think about the death of other people.

PERSONAL PHILOSOPHICAL/RELIGIOUS VIEWS ABOUT DEATH – POTENTIAL IMPACT ON PRACTICE

THE TEMPTATION TO IMPOSE PERSONAL BELIEFS

Fundamentalism has come to be associated with those who hold very strong, perhaps simplistic, religious views and seek to impose those views on everyone else. Such people might impose their views of the meaning of death on people who are dying or, if concerned with ethics, might find it a struggle not to promulgate their ideas. Others, who have come to terms with the thought of their own death, either in religious or philosophical terms, might also be tempted to convince those who are dying that their view is right. This may apply particularly if those who are dying are viewed as struggling to come to terms with what death means to them.

The question of the degree to which we should share our own beliefs with others is a difficult one. Those who are responsible for the care of others need to be aware of the power imbalance implicit in the relationship. The patient may need to feel that the health-care professional has all the answers (at least in relation to treatment), so a variety of views of the helper in this context may carry more weight than if they were expressed outside the helper–patient relationship. The professional helper is usually employed to perform a specific function and this would not normally include evangelism. However, there might be times when the professional is asked a direct question and it is appropriate to give an honest answer. If he or she decides that it is right in response to a direct question to share beliefs, care needs to be taken not to go beyond the question that was asked. It may also be helpful to offer alternative views in addition to one's personal beliefs.

PERSONAL VIEWS AND ANXIETIES AS MEDIATING FACTORS
IN CARING

Moscrop (1995) states, 'It has been noted and mentioned at a recent Royal College of Nursing Cancer Society meeting that those who possess a religious faith can gain an inner strength, which in turn helps them in the care they give to patients and families in distress.' We would draw attention to the word 'can', as religious faith does not necessarily always give inner strength to the helping professional.

The philosophy mentioned earlier of seeing death as the completion of life might result in a focus on issues of unfinished business. Those whose religious or philosophical views have been influenced by Hinduism or Buddhism may also be inclined to think about the end of their own lives in terms of unfinished business. Their treatment of the dying might therefore be affected by that same thinking. As with the example of fundamentalism mentioned above, we need as helping professionals to monitor the extent to which we feel the issue of unfinished business is of concern to the patient and how much it is derived from our own agenda.

If we have never considered our own death and what it means to us, then we are unlikely to be comfortable thinking about death with reference to others. As noted earlier in this chapter, Wilkinson (1991) observed different ways in which nurses block important communication with dying patients. Her research also showed that atheists with the greatest fear of dying were the highest blockers. However, Neimeyer and Van Brunt (1995) found that, while religious belief may result in less death anxiety, those with a moderate level of belief or an ambivalent belief had more problems with death anxiety than atheists or strong believers.

The nature of the belief system of some religious people may also affect their level of death anxiety. For example, in a study by Florian and Kravetz (1983) the fear of personal death scale was administered to 178 Israeli Jews, along with an established measure of religious practice. They found that in highly religious Jews there was a strong anxiety centred on the prospect of punishment in the after life. Such anxiety may also apply for some Moslems and for others in Christian circles, particularly those who come from denominations heavily influenced by Calvinism.

Many helpers who are religious may find comfort in their beliefs in relation to the prospect of imminent death and may unconsciously convey that sense of comfort and lack of fear to those they are caring for. However, others, because of their beliefs about judgement, may convey something of their own anxiety and fear to their patients.

Probably the most important aspect of personal belief systems is to own what we believe or feel and then seek as far as possible to put it to one side. We can then work with patients' own belief systems so that they can maximize any support that they may gain from them.

In this chapter we have considered how fears about death can directly impact on the process of caring. This includes affecting what we say to clients as well as what we don't communicate. We have also discussed how personal belief systems may affect care and that the relationship between the two is not necessarily straightforward. In considering the views of professional helpers about death we noted a wide variability in responses and this suggests that we should not make assumptions about how an individual client may be feeling. Having considered our own thoughts, feelings and beliefs about death, we should then be less likely to project them on to clients. Also, we increase the probability of empathizing with and getting alongside them. The temptation to avoid having meaningful conversations with those who are dying, out of fear of our own concerns being provoked, will be reduced.

The reader may find it helpful to share thoughts on the following questions about death with a colleague. If some of the questions cannot be addressed it would be worth reflecting on why this might be so. For example, is it because of irrational beliefs about tempting fate or a wish to defend oneself against troublesome thoughts? In considering such questions it may also be helpful to keep in mind the point made in Chapter 5 – that preparing for loss can have a beneficial impact on life before loss.

Some personal thoughts to consider about death

- Which of the categories in Table 6.1 reflect your own thoughts about death?
- If you were told that in approximately 6 months time you would die, how would you spend the rest of your life?
- If you were to die soon, what would be a great omission from your life?
- If you knew you would die soon, what would be your most important needs?
- Which three people would you want at your death bed (choose from those who are living now)?
- How does your philosophy of life affect your attitude towards death?
- Would you consider planning your own funeral? (If so, what would it be like?)
- What short epitaph would you like to go on your gravestone or plaque?
- What quality would you not like to be remembered for?
- How could your own thoughts about death affect your ability to work with people who are dying:
- in a helpful way;
- in an unhelpful way?

Understanding the bereavement process

7

Anything that you have, you can lose, anything you are attached to, you can be separated from, anything you love can be taken away from you. Yet, if you really have nothing to lose, you have nothing.

Kalish, 1985

In many ways grief is like falling in love backwards.

Littlewood, 1992

Any serious bereavement impairs the ability to attach meaning to events, and hence to learn from them how to survive.

Marris, 1986

Much has been written about bereavement and it would be difficult to cover all aspects in one chapter. The aim here is, first, to give some information on the subject, so that the reader may have a better understanding of what is happening to his or her client/patient in relation to the bereavement process; second, to help readers who may not have any personal experience of bereavement to see how other experiences of loss can help them to relate to those who are recently bereaved.

In this chapter we will be considering some of the theories that relate to the bereavement process. We will then seek to relate the bereavement process to the reader's own experience of loss. We will go on to examine the concept that being truly present is more important than what is said when seeking to help those who are bereaved. We will then seek to make some suggestions for helping the newly bereaved before, finally, seeking to blend theory and practice in aiding readers in their care of the bereaved.

SOME THEORIES RELATING TO THE BEREAVEMENT PROCESS

There are a number of theories as to what happens in bereavement. We will be outlining some of the most important ones here. We aim to give an overview of the whole process at this point, and towards the end of this section to focus in more detail on the early stages.

Perhaps the most significant contribution to the early thinking on bereavement was the work of John Bowlby (Bowlby, 1979; see also Parkes *et al.*, 1991). In looking at the relationship of parents and children in a clinical situation, Bowlby came to see that the nature of the attachment a child makes with mother or other significant person governs the nature of attachments that are made in later life. Also, the way that the child and mother cope with separation and loss governs the way in which the child will respond to future losses.

In observing what occurred when a mother was forced to leave her child in hospital, Bowlby saw that the child went through various stages in the process of seeking to deal with this situation.

Parkes (1996) has developed the theory in relation to bereavement and has hypothesized four stages in this process:

- **phase 1**: shock, numbness and the pain of grieving;
- **phase 2**: manifestation of fear, guilt, anger and resentment;
- **phase 3**: disengagement, apathy and aimlessness;
- **phase 4**: a gradual hope and a move in new directions.

Parkes sees in bereavement a process not dissimilar to a young child's reaction to the temporary loss of mother or other significant person.

PHASE 1: SHOCK, NUMBNESS AND THE PAIN OF GRIEVING

This initial phase is characterized by shock, and often results in the mourner unconsciously seeking to disbelieve that which they are unable to cope with. Inability to hear what is said about the loved one being dead, or anger at the bearer of bad news, are not unusual responses to hearing the news that someone has died. (We will be looking at this in more detail later.)

This pattern of shock is accompanied by numbness, a 'going through the motions' with no emotional involvement. This process may continue until after the funeral, and usually lasts a week or two.

Between the death and the funeral there are many practical arrangements that have to be made and administrative tasks that have to be accomplished. Often this is done by the bereaved person appearing almost to be acting on automatic pilot.

This is followed by pangs of grief. The experience is not one of continuous severity, but an experience of waves of acute emotional pain that threaten to overwhelm and destroy the bereaved but somehow do not.

PHASE 2: MANIFESTATION OF FEAR, GUILT AND ANGER

In this phase, there are often manifestations of fear. 'If it could happen to him it could happen to me.' Often the bereaved will find themselves having the same physical symptoms as the last illness of the one they loved. In the situation where a partner died in his or her sleep there may be a fear of not waking up.

Guilt is common in this stage, and shows itself in the often asked questions, 'What did I do wrong?' and, 'Should I have done more?' The many, 'if only's', the recently bereaved are often heard to say can also be an indication of guilt.

Anger and resentment, which may be felt towards the person who has died – 'How could you leave me?' – are often not acceptable feelings to the mourner, and that anger can then be projected on to the professional carers or on to relatives.

PHASE 3: DISENGAGEMENT, APATHY AND AIMLESSNESS

The bereaved person reaches a phase that marks the stage of no-man's-land, when he or she is beginning to accept the finality of death but is not yet ready to re-invest energy into other things. The resultant experience is one of apathy and aimlessness. 'I don't know who I am any more' is often heard at this time.

PHASE 4: A GRADUAL HOPE AND A MOVE IN NEW DIRECTIONS

Finally, in this stage there is a return to hope on the part of mourners, and a move towards reinvesting themselves into other activities. In the case of the loss of a partner this is a period of finding out who I am, now that I am no longer a partner. New relationships may be entered into and an active social life may begin to emerge. Also, new interests may be found or old ones rediscovered. It begins to feel as if life is not over and a new phase can begin.

Hopson (1981), as discussed in Chapter 1, has outlined a theory of change, which, though not specifically dealing with bereavement, necessarily incorporates it. This theory follows a similar pattern to the one discussed above. In Hopson's theory there are seven stages in the process of change. This model may be seen as complementary to that of Parkes.

Hopson's important contribution here, however, is to relate this pattern of dealing with change to all experiences of loss and not only to bereavement. As we will see later, this idea helps us to be able to relate to those who are bereaved, even if we have not experienced a major bereavement ourselves.

If the reader is one who prefers to have things presented visually rather than in written form, then Wilson's (1993) 'whirlpool of grief' (Figure 7.1) may be helpful.

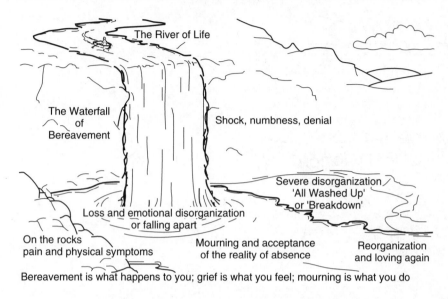

The River of Life

The Waterfall of Bereavement

Shock, numbness, denial

Severe disorganization, 'All Washed Up' or 'Breakdown'

Loss and emotional disorganization or falling apart

On the rocks pain and physical symptoms

Mourning and acceptance of the reality of absence

Reorganization and loving again

Bereavement is what happens to you; grief is what you feel; mourning is what you do

Figure 7.1   The whirlpool of grief (source: Richard Wilson, Kingston Hospital).

As can be seen, it includes the same elements of the bereavement process. Coming down, the waterfall represents a sudden disruption to one's life, which may have been flowing along quite smoothly up to this point. It represents shock and numbness. The whirlpool represents the emotional upheaval and disorganization that follows (anger, guilt, anxiety, etc.). Being 'all washed up' on the banks of the river could represent 'being stuck' and unable to move on. Before being able to progress one would have to get back into the whirlpool and experience the emotional turmoil. With gradual acceptance of the loss, one would be able to move along the river of life again.

Another pictorial model is that of the grief wheel (Figure 7.2).

If one imagines various aspects (or functions) of one's life, such as being a worker or a parent, then these can be disrupted by a loss. Life will not go on as normal and one will have to work round the wheel of grief. Protest (anger, yearning, searching, etc.) and disorganization (aimlessness, hopelessness, loss of confidence) are equivalent to the whirlpool in Wilson's model. With reorganization one can go along the road of life again and be able to fulfil various life roles.

The last model presented in this chapter is that of William Worden (1991), already mentioned in Chapter 1 in relation to redundancy. Worden, like Parkes, also has stages of grief and the headings he gives are in fact very similar to Parkes'. Where Worden differs from Parkes is that, rather than referring to grief stages, Worden uses the term 'tasks'.

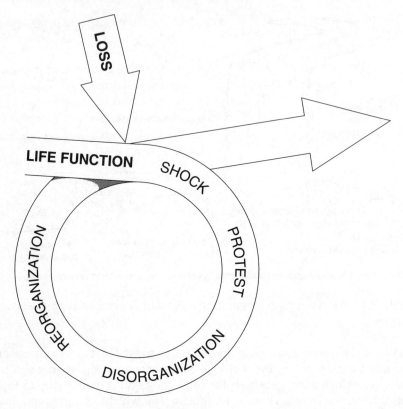

Figure 7.2 The grief wheel (reproduced from Goodall *et al.*, 1994, with permission).

He talks of 'tasks of mourning' that have to be accomplished for equilibrium to be re-established.

This task perspective can be very helpful. Parkes' stages can imply that the process goes on entirely independently of the bereaved person's control. In contrast Worden's view is that the bereaved person moves from stage to stage as he or she fulfils the tasks required for effective grieving.

This idea of tasks that have to be accomplished before mourning can move to the next stage is illustrated in the following anecdote. In the days of coal fires, the coal man would often drop the coal in a place from where it had to be shovelled into the coal bin. This work could be done in different ways. For example, the person shovelling could put his or her back into the work and clear it quickly, or s/he could take frequent rests, do the job as effectively, but take longer over it. In the same way, in the authors' observation, the tasks of mourning can be accomplished either over a shorter and more intense period, or over a longer period with, seemingly, a less intense experience of grief. It would appear that there is a negative correlation between the level of distress in the grief process and the time the grieving takes. Whatever the time frame, there is still a finite quantity of grief to be worked through in the same way that there is a finite quantity of coal in the analogy.

The importance of enabling such grief work is stressed by Stroebe and Stroebe (1987): 'The major task . . . is to encourage grief work . . . being able to talk over the loss, to be able to identify and express feelings of grief, helps the bereaved to come to terms with the death and to ultimately make a better adjustment.'

All the authors quoted so far appear to express the bereavement process in terms of some sort of linear progression. There are, however, those who feel that this hypothesis is rather too tidy and that bereavement is in fact much more 'messy'.

Littlewood (1993), quoting Kastenbaum and Germain, considers that seeing bereavement in this tidy fashion causes any deviation to be labelled abnormal. She goes on to say that the experiences of grief 'are better characterized in terms of wave after wave of violently contradictory emotional impulses'. Littlewood also suggests that the theories we have outlined present grief in a culturally acceptable way. Spiegel (1977) points out that all that has been said in the above applies very much to a Western society in which church rituals and local customs have all but disappeared.

Wortman and Silver (1989) question whether the experiences of grief outlined by these theories are in fact universally experienced. They argue that not everyone goes through periods of depression, or even that distress is part of everyone's experience of loss. Like Procrustes in Greek mythology, who had a guest bed in which those who were too short were stretched to fit and those too long were cut down, Wortman and Silver (1989) question whether there is a tendency in these models to try to make everyone fit. Those who do not are then in danger of being labelled pathological in their grieving.

In fairness to Parkes and Worden, they recognize the limitations of their stages or tasks and they speak of them very much in terms of working models rather than fixed laws. The authors find it helpful to look at bereavement in terms of overall progression towards adjustment, recognizing, however, that progress is often that of the tide coming in, ebbing and flowing but all the time coming higher up the beach, rather than a constant progression from one stage/task to another.

Before we turn to look at the early stages of grieving in more detail, it might be helpful to point out that those who are dying go through a similar experience as they seek to come to terms with the imminence of their own death. We will be dealing with this later, in Chapter 8.

So we have seen that, in general terms, grief follows a pattern that can be mapped. The end of this journey may for some be a complete recovery. They may end up significantly more whole people than when they started. Those who have lost a partner may find another equally satisfying, if different, relationship as the one whose passing caused them so much pain. Others will never completely recover. As one of the authors often puts it, 'For some, it can be like losing a leg. You may learn to walk again, but it will never be as it was when you had two legs.'

THE EARLY STAGES OF GRIEF

Some professional helpers will be concerned with what happens at the time of death and soon after. In Parkes' model (1996) the first stage is that of shock. In Worden's (1991) it is the task of accepting the reality of loss, while for Hopson the first stage is immobilization and the second is minimization (a desperate desire or attempt to make the event less important).

All these descriptions imply that it is actually an incredibly difficult thing to acknowledge that someone who is very close has died. They suggest that the inner world of the bereaved has been blown apart. Mourners speak of 'a gaping hole that has been left' or of having been 'torn apart', to express the magnitude of what has happened to them.

The response to the realization of such a loss is the taking up of fairly extreme coping mechanisms. Listed below are some of the common responses in the immediate post-bereavement stage.

- **Shock**: this includes physical symptoms. 'Pulse and respirations are increased . . . The patient often shows signs of restlessness and anxiety . . . There also may be weakness, lethargy, pallor and a cool moist skin' (Mosby, 1994).
- **Denial and disbelief**: this may be a deliberate refusal to believe what is being said, as expressed in the phrase, 'I don't believe you'. Alternatively, there may a failure to register what is being said and this can be viewed as a form of unconscious denial.
- **Anger**: this could be at the person (bearer of the bad news) who dares to destroy their internal world, at the one who has died, or at those they feel ought to have prevented their loved one's death.
- **Sadness**: sometimes this seems overwhelming. It is often expressed in uncontrollable tears, screaming or keening (a stylized form of wailing, dependent on the cultural norms of the person who is bereaved).

Many of these symptoms are reported in an article written by William Wharton in the *Sunday Times Magazine* (1994), which is itself taken from William Wharton's book *Wrongful Deaths*. The article tells the harrowing story of how William and his wife Rosemary hear the news that their daughter, son-in-law and two granddaughters were killed in a freak accident on an Oregon highway caused by stubble burning in an adjacent field. When he returns from cycling, William is given the news by his wife Rosemary, who begins to cry. He relates, 'I hold her tighter. I'm beginning to shiver. I feel cold all the way inside myself.'

He describes what happened the next morning, as he got out of bed.

> Then I stand up. Immediately it's as if I am struck hard in the back from behind. I fall to my knees. As I land, my hands are in fists on the worn shag rug. It's as if I've been knocked down in a football game, clipped. I catch my breath for several seconds. Then I can, and begin to sob with such violence I almost throw up. I fight for breath between sobs ...

Fortunately, for most people the experience of being bereaved is not as sudden, or as violent, as it was for the Whartons (though sudden and violent deaths are not uncommon). Also, the reaction of those hearing about the loss of someone they love may differ markedly from that of the Whartons. Each person reacts in their own individual way. Nevertheless, the reactions described above are not untypical.

RELATING THE BEREAVEMENT PROCESS TO OUR OWN EXPERIENCE OF LOSS

Every person's experience of grief is unique. As carers we are never in a position to say that we know how mourners are feeling. Their journey through grief is essentially their own private path. No one else can walk in their steps. Nevertheless we may be able to accompany them for a short distance and in so doing help to share the load.

If we have experienced a major loss ourselves, and have integrated the loss so that others' grief does not trigger our own, we may feel more comfortable in dealing with the bereaved than those who have not had such an experience. If, on the other hand, we are still feeling our own loss sharply, we may find it very much more difficult.

With life expectancy continually increasing, most of us today do not experience a major loss until we are well into our forties; some even later than that. For such people, bereavement poses major problems of relating to mourners in their experience of loss.

In this situation it is helpful to be aware that bereavement is only one end of a continuum of loss (as discussed in Chapter 2). The process by which we come to terms with any loss is basically the same. The difference is only that of degree. Penson (1990) states that the word bereavement means 'to be robbed of something valued'. While that is especially true of bereavement, it is also true of many other lesser situations that we are all likely to experience at some time. This could be the loss of a favourite pet, a lost article, the break-up of a relationship or the experience of being robbed or burgled. Traumatic experiences such as amputation, mastectomy or hysterectomy, rape or divorce come much closer to the experience of bereavement for many in the continuum of loss. The reader may find it helpful to think about his or her own experience of loss in general, in relation to some of the models discussed earlier. This may help to give insight into the experiences of the bereaved. It is important that we should be able to do this, at least to some degree. If we do not, we stand completely out of the field of the bereaved person's experience. If this is the case, we may be able to offer physical aid but will be unable to help the bereaved person in their distress.

BEING TRULY PRESENT PLAYS A MORE IMPORTANT ROLE IN BEREAVEMENT SUPPORT THAN WHAT WE SAY

Perhaps the most important thing that can be said in this section is that there are no right words to say. There is nothing that anyone can say that will make it right, or make it better. Often just being there with the bereaved is more valuable than anything we might say. What is said is often forgotten anyway, but the sense of 'presence' may be treasured for a long time. A touch of a hand or an expression of care can often be more powerful than a whole host of words. Having said that, we will be dealing in Chapter 14 with basic counselling techniques and highlighting some things not to say.

It has been said of Job's comforters in the Bible that they were a great help to Job in expressing their sorrow at his loss and sitting with him. Unfortunately, they went down in history as the wrong kind of example when they started to open their mouths and say all the wrong things!

Bayly (1969), discussing his own experience of bereavement within a Christian perspective of death, writes:

> I was sitting, torn by grief. Someone came and talked to me of God's dealings, of why it happened, of hope beyond the grave. He talked constantly, he said things I knew were true. I was unmoved, except to wish he'd go away. He finally did. Another came and sat beside me. He didn't talk. He didn't ask leading questions. He just sat beside me for an hour and more, listened when I said something, answered briefly, prayed simply, left. I was moved. I was comforted. I hated to see him go.

It might be thought that this example is rather extreme. Remaining silent, or virtually so, is not necessarily the answer to dealing with people who have been bereaved. What is important is to be real and to acknowledge to the mourners, and to ourselves, that we do not have all the answers. In addition, we might find it helpful to say to ourselves that it is OK not to have all the answers because no one has.

Parkes (1996) encourages carers to show their feelings in this context and says that if helpers are ashamed, or feel destroyed by their feelings, they will be of no help to the newly bereaved and had better stay out of the way!

We need to be real in the sense of showing that we are not automatons. This includes conveying that what has happened, and is happening, is distressing to us as well as to the relatives, and also being sensitive and responsive to the needs of the bereaved without being officious. These are the things that are most helpful in a situation where someone has lost a person he or she cares for. There are, however, certain practical considerations that may ease the way for the relative or friend.

SOME SUGGESTIONS FOR HELPING THE NEWLY BEREAVED

We have talked about the expression of feelings on the part of the helper or carer. But what about those of the mourner? Free expression of emotion is not generally acceptable in our society (except, it seems, at a football match!). There may be times when it is necessary to control the emotional display of the recently bereaved. Breaking or throwing of furniture, for instance, would not be conceived by most people as being acceptable. On the other hand, helpers should not be too ready to try to prevent the expression of strong emotion, providing that it will not do damage to the mourner or to anyone else. In such circumstances, the answer may be to take mourners to another room rather than to try to stop them from expressing their grief. Parkes (1996) has written that there is an optimal level of grieving for each individual and that it is important for those feelings to be allowed expression. For more information on this see Chapter 13.

Beriman (1991) quotes Herman Melville:

Tears unwashed are stones upon the heart
that choke the healing stream.

She also quotes Shakespeare:

Give sorrow words: the grief that does not speak
Whispers the o'er-fraught heart, and bids it break.

Macbeth Act IV Scene 3

Those who grieve should also be given the opportunity to view the body if they so wish. For some this is extremely helpful in coming to terms with the fact that the person has died. Others, however, find it very traumatic and unhelpful. By being given the choice, the bereaved can make their own decision as to whether or not it would be helpful to them. But what about when the deceased is badly disfigured, by an accident for instance? Wright (1989) suggests that in such cases there is often a recognizable part of the person free from injury that can be viewed, touched or held. It may be that a crushed skull can be bandaged to reveal only the unmutilated face. Or a hand with a particular ring can be held where the rest of the body would be too distressing to view. We must be careful not to add to the relatives' distress by letting them see things that might magnify their notions of the patient's sufferings before death.

Wright (1989), writing in the context of Emergency Department work, refers to the loss of autonomy that people experience in hospital. 'One elderly lady (and she was not alone) told how she was pleased when the nurse said she may have things to say to her dead husband, even if it was only goodbye. She was not sure how it would appear, being seen talking to somebody dead, or whether she would have been overheard.'

Wright (1989) also notes, 'Another said: "It was nice that the nurse touched his hand and said I could do the same. When you have laid them out (is that what you call it?) you are not sure if you are allowed to touch them . . ." At this time we must support and facilitate those experiences which will bring comfort and will usefully begin that process we call grief.'

All that we have written about the value of viewing the body is irrelevant if there is no body to view. Unfortunately, there are times when it seems clear that someone has died but no body can be found. This is the case in certain murder cases, but it can also be true of people who are lost at sea or who have died in a severe fire or as a result of war. There are particular problems for those who are left behind in accepting the fact of death when there is no body. There are also problems with not having the focus for grief that a body gives.

In Chapter 10, we will deal with issues such as 'last rites' and prayers for the sick. At this point it is helpful merely to note that such a service may be of help and consolation for those who are at a loss as to how to say goodbye.

The authors have also found that wives and husbands in long-term psychiatric care may not, on being widowed, be able to attend the funeral of their partner. In such cases it may be very helpful to hold a memorial service on the ward, with perhaps a photograph of the dead person in place of the coffin. This can be a simple service using some of the readings and prayers that were or are at that time being said in the actual funeral service.

There are special problems when the loss is that of an unborn child. We call those born dead 'stillbirths' or 'fetuses' and in so doing emotionally distance ourselves from them. To the parents it is their child. Taking a photograph of the child who is stillborn or who has died shortly after death and offering it to the parents can be a great help to their grieving. It is important that such photographs be taken before any post-mortem and prior to the body becoming discoloured. Some hospitals keep such photographs for up to 3 months after the death in case the parents, having initially declined, then make a request to have them. An alternative or addition to photographs is foot- and hand-prints of the child. Other hospitals keep a written record of all those who have been born and named but have died so that a memorial to that lost potential is kept. We have written earlier about the importance of viewing the body. This may be particularly important for parents, who may have a great need to hold their dead baby.

There are particular problems for those who have suffered miscarriage and even induced abortions. These can often be treated as non-events resulting in the deaths of non-persons, but for the mother, and often for the father too, the unborn child may have gained the status of personhood (Stewart and Dent, 1994).

Cot deaths also are a cause of great distress for parents. This is often accompanied by severe guilt feelings. The 'if onlys' that often accompany death can be greatly magnified in cot deaths.

Neither must we forget that among those who grieve are children. They may not be able to express their loss as eloquently as adults but they feel it just as much. In particular, we must be aware of the tendency for children to engage in 'magical thinking'. Jewett (1994) writes, 'Younger children perceive they are the centre of the universe. His own thoughts, wishes, and actions, the child believes, cause what happens to himself and to other people.' Magical thinking is never completely eradicated in any of us, and it tends to recur in times of crisis, even in adults (e.g. 'If only I had a new job everything would be fine', 'If only I had insisted he stay home, it wouldn't have happened'). Jewett (1994) relates how a 5-year-old developed an acute fear of closets. This fear was not related to obvious fears such as a fear of the dark, of monsters lurking or of being trapped. It arose out of overhearing a remark that 'someone had come out of the closet and had AIDS'. His reasoning suggested that anyone who entered a closet was in danger of catching AIDS and dying from it. Magical thinking is a particular concern when related to guilt. Here it is the tendency to think that unrelated behaviour may somehow be a cause of death.

Above all we must give time and space to the bereaved to make their farewell in their own way and at their own pace. Chaplains can be of great help here when urgent duties call others away to do other things.

SEEKING TO BLEND THEORY AND PRACTICE

The unknown is a great fear. On early maps notes were to be found in the seas around the coast at points beyond which sailors were afraid to go. The mottos often read, 'Here be monsters'. Uncharted territory has its own terror of monsters lurking. To know something of what is occurring in the minds and emotions of those who have been bereaved can give us at least some sense of being in control. We hope that what has been written in this chapter will provide a foundation for such a knowledge.

Another important issue in dealing with the bereaved is the assurance that we do not have to 'get it right'. Often simply being ourselves, allowing the bereaved to express what they are feeling and supporting them in their pain, is all that is needed and will be remembered for a long time with gratitude by those who receive it. More will be said on the practicalities of this in Chapter 12.

The most important thing to remember in this whole area is that we cannot make grieving painless. We cannot heal the broken heart, we can only facilitate a good beginning to the long road that is recovery from grief.

Maureen Lahiff (1994), formerly Professor of Nursing and Midwifery, resigned her post following the death of her son David when he was only 20. She writes:

> Among the key things I learnt were that the first 2 years, give or take a few weeks, is the **acute** phase. What a relief! Wherever did professional carers get the idea that from 12 months after the event we (the bereaved parents) should be 'back to normal'? There is no normality as we knew it – only a recreated life, one in which a deep scar remains, however well or poorly it is healed.

These observations should not create despair in helping professionals. It is a great privilege to help at any stage in the process of grief. Whatever the final outcome we can, and often do, affect the process for good.

As was stated at the beginning of this chapter, there has been a lot written about bereavement. We have given an overview of the bereavement process with reference to some of the major theories. We have also sought to assist readers in relating their own experience of loss to the bereavement process and to feel more comfortable in their dealings with the bereaved.

Understanding the dying person and the effects on relatives and ourselves

8

*They make me mad when they come in here and tell me what's happening on **my** unit. Sooner or later they go back to work, and take over what I want to be doing. I have to lie here in this stupid hospital and die!*

Nurse dying of breast cancer at 32,
quoted in Callanan and Kelley, 1992

I think a good death is not being in pain, feeling fulfilled with your life, feeling as if you've done everything that you needed to do and that all your house is in order.

Nurse

I'm not afraid to die but I'm afraid of the manner in which I die. I wouldn't like to lose my dignity and I hate pain.

Hospice worker

Some relatives are very hard to deal with in as much as they don't accept from the word go that the patient is dying.

Nurse

As we tend not to talk about death and dying, we do not have the opportunity to compare our own views with those of colleagues, family or friends. This can lead to ambivalence or confusion, for example, about what constitutes a 'good death'. In this chapter we will consider how such uncertainty can impact on our ability to understand what a dying person may be experiencing, and how the death of a patient can affect us and those who have known him/her, particularly relatives. (The impact of the death of a patient on other patients will be discussed in Chapter 9.) Firstly, however, some views on common emotional processes in dying people will be discussed.

Probably the most well known description of responses to dying is that provided by Kübler-Ross (1969). She talks of five stages, the first being **denial**, in which individuals just cannot accept that they have a life-threatening illness. Although writing in relation to bereavement, the initial section of Grollman's (1995) description of denial also aptly depicts its occurrence in the process of dying:

> 'Oh, dear God, it isn't true.
> Not to me!
> There must be some mistake.'

Kübler-Ross's (1969) next stage is **anger**, often characterized by 'Why should this happen to me?' The anger could be directed, for example, at a doctor for not diagnosing the problem earlier when a cure might have been a possibility. It may be directed at oneself for previous unhealthy behaviour such as smoking. Frustration and anger are closely connected and the frustration of not being able to complete dearly held plans, for example, can result in extreme anger. There may be envy and resentment at others who are going about their daily life, active and healthy.

Bargaining is perhaps the least well understood stage because it is a response to dying that is not talked about in relation to bereavement (many of the responses to dying, such as the denial and anger already mentioned, are also experienced in bereavement – see Chapter 7). It is referred to as the 'Yes me, but . . .' stage. The dying person is trying to change the inevitable outcome by a process of cognitive negotiation. The aim is usually to get more time. An example might be a dialogue with God: 'I'll be good, I'll even be nice to people who I can't really stand, if I can just live another 3 months until my daughter's wedding.'

Callanan and Kelley (1992) present a useful analogy for helping to understand bargaining. Children at bedtime may negotiate for extra time by asking for just one more story or to be allowed to stay up a little later to watch a television programme. Their side of the bargain might be, for example, to be good, to definitely go to sleep after the extended time or do an extra household chore the next day.

Depression (the fourth stage) may be associated with fear of dying and the prospect of having to leave loved ones behind. It will probably also be connected with (1) losses that have already been experienced such as loss of independence or usual role within the family and (2) loss of plans or hopes such as an unfulfilled ambition to visit a particular place or to see one's first grandchild. (These are the 'loss of oughts' referred to in Chapter 4.) Feelings of depression may also result from a realization that bargaining is not going to work.

Acceptance can be described as a stage which is often empty or void of all emotion and Samarel refers to this as 'signifying the end of the struggle'. Ward (1993) refers to this stage as involving a gradual process of withdrawing in which patients want to see fewer people and may prefer those that do visit to sit with them quietly. Although not talked about in relation to the model, some people clearly can have a serene and halcyon death. One nurse described her experience of nursing a 94-year-old lady who died in hospital:

> This lady had never been in hospital in her life and she died of cancer. I'm not sure if anybody had ever told her that she was going to die but she had this serene quality about her of complete acceptance of what was happening to her ... It was almost like a halo, it was lovely to look at and sit with her.

As with bereavement reactions, people do not experience these emotions in a neat order or necessarily one at a time. Kübler-Ross herself stated that progression through the various stages is not necessarily linear and may not be rushed; in addition, that not all people experience all stages.

It should be noted that, although many of these stages can be observed in dying people, the theory has never really been tested out. Consequently, it should not be applied in a literal sense, for example, expecting or encouraging patients to move from one stage to the next. Corr (1993) pointed out that there is a wide variation in how individuals cope with dying. Such a general theory takes no account of the many factors that may affect how a particular person deals with dying. These could include previous ways of coping with crises, general personality, views on religious or spiritual matters, ability to cope with pain, unresolved relationship difficulties and his or her social and physical environment. The danger of having a theory that leads us into thinking that we understand individual dying patients is that we may not take the trouble to find out their particular holistic needs.

Another way of trying to understand the process of dying is described by Glaser and Strauss (1968). They use the term 'dying trajectory' to categorize various types of death in relation to time. A lingering trajectory is when there is a gradual decline over a long period; an example of this might be someone with Alzheimer's disease who is in residential care. The expected quick trajectory is when the patient has an illness that is likely to lead to death in the near future. The unexpected quick trajectory is when a patient suddenly deteriorates and dies for no immediately obvious reason. Various combinations of 'certainty' and time constitute different types of dying trajectory. An example is certain death at a known time, e.g. some types of late-diagnosed cancer. Samarel (1995) points out that the way dying trajectories are perceived is important because it can result in hopelessness or high levels of anxiety even though the perceived expectations may not be accurate.

Glaser and Strauss (1965) also described different types of awareness in dying people and those around them, which can affect the quality of communication between all concerned. These will be discussed in Chapter 11.

PROFESSIONAL AMBIVALENCE ABOUT A GOOD DEATH

If professional helpers have clear views about what they would want to die of and what constitutes a good or appropriate death, shouldn't this help them to understand dying patients? It is the view of the authors that this is not necessarily the case because in workshops we have run there are often widely varying views and inconsistencies. One exercise (developed by two psychologists, Glyn Owens and Gus Baker – personal communication) involves ranking a list of possible causes of death, giving rank 1 to the cause of death you would prefer for yourself, rank 2 to the next preferred and so on. Table 8.1 gives the accumulated results of conducting this exercise with various groups of helping professionals, including nurses, doctors (house officers) and clinical psychology trainees (the sum of the rank frequencies in each row are not necessarily the same as some people do not rank every illness). It helps when completing this exercise to know something about the various illnesses; for instance, pain may be a particular problem in lung cancer and cancer of the pancreas and the 5-year survival rates for these two diseases is very low (of the order of 5–10%), and Alzheimer's disease involves gradual deterioration.

It will be noted that the most commonly preferred cause of death is heart attack and the second most preferred is stroke. The two least preferred causes of death were multiple sclerosis and Alzheimer's disease. Table 8.2 represents the factors that were being considered in making the rankings in Table 8.1. The most important factor was given rank 1, the second most important rank 2 and so on.

It can be seen that time course (brief versus prolonged) was the factor that most people had in mind when judging their preferred cause of death and pain was the second most important factor. This correlates with the choice of a quick death from a heart attack or stroke.

Table 8.1 Own cause of death preferences in helping professionals

Ranking	1	2	3	4	5	6	7	8	9	10
Lung cancer	2	0	5	4	9	12	13	10	4	4
Malignant melanoma	1	8	4	13	13	13	3	6	3	0
Heart attack	60	9	4	1	1	0	0	1	0	0
Breast cancer	3	3	3	13	8	10	10	8	3	1
Alzheimer's disease	4	4	4	5	3	3	4	3	12	28
Cancer of pancreas	0	7	18	8	8	10	7	2	3	2
Stroke	6	39	10	1	2	2	4	2	6	1
Stomach cancer	1	1	5	10	11	8	5	14	4	4
Multiple sclerosis	0	0	4	10	2	2	2	7	20	24
Oesophageal cancer	0	1	6	4	8	3	16	12	11	6

Table 8.2 Reasons for deciding own cause of death preferences in health professionals

Ranking	1	2	3	4	5	6	7	8	9
Pain	18	21	10	4	3	7	6	1	7
Time course	37	14	9	7	7	2	1	1	1
Whether cancer	4	1	6	1	7	7	13	20	15
Whether would involve surgery	0	2	1	4	0	11	10	20	24
Dependence on others	2	12	10	11	12	8	10	11	2
Physical deterioration	2	8	7	18	15	14	9	0	6
Uncertainty	3	0	9	4	11	11	17	11	7
Loss of personal dignity	14	6	10	14	14	8	3	5	4
Mental deterioration	7	9	11	13	8	8	8	4	7

Another observation from the results of these exercises is that there is also considerable variation in the rankings of possible causes of death and the reasons for these choices. This applies even within the same professional group. One conclusion from this is that, if such variation exists among professionals who have a lot in common, e.g. interest in helping and educational level, then the variation among patients will be even greater. Hence it is unwise to make assumptions about how individuals may be viewing their illness and eventual death.

Often in workshops the authors have conducted the following simple exercise immediately following the one above – to ask the group to brainstorm what constitutes a good death. As the exercises follow one another it is highly unlikely that participants will have forgotten their ratings in the first one. Table 8.3 represents combined views on a good death over a number of workshops, so any one individual could believe that a particular combination of these ideas constitutes a good death.

These perceptions are very similar to those of a group of 20 health professionals in a palliative care unit who, in a study by Payne et al. (1996), were asked what they thought constituted a 'good' death. They also have some similarities to the views of Nimock et al. (1987), who described the 'goodness' of a death in terms of the degree of acceptance among those involved, the level of mutual support, mitigation of discomfort and isolation and the completion of unfinished business. The reader familiar with Maslow's (1987) hierarchy of human needs will recognize that the needs at death given in Table 8.3 are very similar to needs in life. Maslow (1987) describes, for instance, physiological and safety needs, the need for love and a sense of belonging, the search for meaning and self-actualization. It will be noted that the ideas on a good death include having time to discuss life after you've gone, dealing with unfinished business in one's relationships and being able to say goodbye. It is at this point that the ambivalence and incoherence in views

Table 8.3 Some thoughts of health professionals on what is a good death

Pain/symptom control	• Pain-free/Good symptom control
No 'excess' medical intervention	• No/minimal medical intervention • Not having inappropriate treatment
Physical environment	• Comfort and warmth • Peaceful and quiet/Calm environment • Privacy
Understanding/information	• Having information and understanding condition • Understanding of illness by relatives
Practical matters	• Practical help/Enough time to discuss life after you've gone • Organized/prepared, e.g. having a will, insurance, money for funeral
Social environment	• Support/Listening time • Open communication/Everybody knows what's going on • Involve family • Positive attitude among carers • Relatives not 'moving in'
Participation/choice/control	• Having people you want there/Family present or not – patient's wish • Choose surroundings/Choose where to die • Involved in planning, e.g. to donate organs if patient wishes
Dealing with unfinished business	• Relationships left in order • Things not left unsaid
Psychological/spiritual	• Having time to prepare, e.g. organize own funeral • Dignity/Acceptance • Completion/Memories/Perception of a fulfilled life • Spiritual needs met, e.g. last rites • Belief/Spiritual step – enlightenment • Being able to say goodbye/Someone close present
Timing/Nature of death	• Die in sleep/Pain-free/Not to know • Timely/Not unduly prolonged • Everything possible been done

about death and dying become apparent. Achieving such goals is not possible if one's death is quick and sudden, as in the case of suffering a heart attack.

It is possible that people are compartmentalizing their thinking, so that, when asked to choose a preferred cause of their own death, they think purely selfishly in terms of what would cause them the least suffering. These choices may be motivated by fear, for example of pain and progressive deterioration. In contrast, when asked to think generally about a good death, wider practical, psychological and spiritual issues are considered, probably from the perspective of the dying person (somebody else) and his/her relatives.

The implications of these observations can be summarized as follows:

- If we project our own fears about death on patients, this may interfere with our ability to care effectively. This may apply particularly if the dying person is in pain or in a 'lingering trajectory.'
- Because of the wide variation in people's views about death and dying we should not make assumptions about what an individual dying person may be thinking or feeling.
- Our individual conceptions of a good death may be limited and so we may not be aware of some other factors that could be important to an individual patient. The quote at the beginning of this chapter was one nurse's understanding of a good death. Another nurse stated, 'I think dying people need freedom from pain, maintenance of dignity, somebody to talk to, somebody sometimes just to sit beside them, just someone there.' This might lead to focusing on these areas in preference to many other issues, such as those illustrated in Table 8.3.

EFFECTS ON RELATIVES

The way that relatives react may be affected by various factors, for example their personality, the degree of intimacy in the relationship with the patient, the way they perceive they have been treated by the medical profession and their level of understanding about the patient's illness.

Some relatives will experience anticipatory grief: in other words, rather than beginning to feel grief after the patient's death the emotions begin before the patient has died. This is particularly likely to occur if there is a change in the personality of the dying person. Littlewood (1992) quotes an example of a woman in her 50s whose father suffered from senile dementia. When he was admitted to residential care, this woman felt that her father 'was as good as dead'. She reported that she experienced little reaction to the news of his death. Sometimes having a relative who is no longer the person you knew can be very distressing.

A woman in her 70s whose husband had a major stroke told one of the authors that 'it was worse than if he had died'. This man was in hospital and could not speak or really do anything for himself.

While such anticipatory grieving may be helpful to the relative, it could be to the detriment of the dying patient, who may feel abandoned. The opposite situation applies if, in the process of caring for the dying person, the relative becomes totally enmeshed in this role. In this scenario the relative may lose previous social contacts and so eventually find it more difficult to adjust to bereavement. In contrast, the patient may benefit from the extra attention.

Callanan and Kelly (1992) illustrate how, when the dying patient begins to accept death, this can be more difficult for the relative. A man dying from cancer hardly spoke in his last days of life, and seemed to be comfortable and at peace. His wife felt rejected; 'It's like he's going and he's happy to be going and I can't stand it.'

Sometimes relatives who cannot accept that the patient is dying may feel that staff are not trying their best and wonder whether they should try another place and another treatment. When they visit and notice a physical deterioration in the patient, they may blame the nurses or doctors.

Another problem for staff can arise when relatives promise to be with the dying person at the end. A hospice nurse described her experience: 'They don't want to go away and they can sit for days ... And then if you do send them away or let them go or give them permission to leave and the patient dies and they're not there, you feel guilty because they've not fulfilled their roles.' It is perhaps worth noting at this point that a few nurses have mentioned to the authors their experience of patients dying soon after relatives have left the bedside. This anecdotal evidence suggests that some patients may wait for their relatives to leave because it is easier for them to die without loved ones present. An example of what the above nurse might say to a relative who is feeling guilty about not being there is: 'Well, look, you were here on Sunday, you had a lovely day, you went round the garden, that was the time he must have decided (to die).'

Some relatives have misconceptions that may make them very anxious about being present at the patient's death. One example of this is the belief that patients with cancer of the lung will bleed to death or 'cough up their lungs'. Clearly, there is a useful role here for the nurse or doctor to provide accurate information. Another application of this educational role would be with, for example, the relative who once said to a nurse that all patients with cancer had to be cremated as it was the law.

A general nurse made a comment in relation to relatives that echoes an earlier theme in this chapter, about not making assumptions:

'I've learnt not to prejudge how a relative is going to behave. When the actual death occurs, I take things one step at a time because you're never sure who you're going to be supporting.'

In this section we have only explored some of the issues that affect relatives when a patient is dying and the interaction between patient and relative. The reader may wish to consider other aspects of loss for relatives, which space does not allow us to consider here. These might include, for example, guilt if the patient cannot be cared for at home and the possible loss of a sexual relationship. For more on working with relatives see, for example, Brewin and Sparshott, 1996. The complex issue of collusion, which results in poor communication between relative and patient, will be discussed in Chapter 11.

EFFECTS ON OURSELVES

Caring for dying people can evoke difficult issues for helping professionals, some of which have been referred to in earlier chapters; for example, difficulties with the thought of being dependent on others. Maguire (1985) observed that doctors and nurses involved in terminal care use distancing tactics to avoid patients' emotional suffering. For example, they make assumptions about why patients are upset ('You are bound to be upset with getting so much pain. We'll up your pain killers.'). The reasons for such behaviour may include a fear of unleashing strong emotions or of being overwhelmed by the patient's suffering and loss. Getting too close to patients would, for example, make it harder to accept that they could not always guarantee them a peaceful death. Lev (1989) also describes avoidance behaviours by physicians and nurses and suggests that this could be due to reminders of the limitations of professional care and the fact that control over one's fate may be an illusion. The latter point relates to being reminded of one's own mortality. Interestingly, on some hospital wards, dying people may be moved to a side room and rational arguments can be presented for this – for example, there is more privacy when relatives visit. However, such a move probably means that nursing staff will have less contact with the patient. Is this, in effect, another distancing tactic?

Saunders and Valente (1994) suggest that nurses may question the dignity, preventability and appropriateness of a death and also that self-examination may include asking questions such as: 'Did I do enough?' and 'Should I have done (or not done) something to help reduce suffering or improve quality of life'. The theme of feeling that they had 'let a patient down' emerged from some of the authors' interviews with nurses.

This comment is from a nurse who had identified with and had a good relationship with a patient: 'I felt I'd let her down because she'd asked to go home and die in her own bed . . . I can remember sitting at the office desk and I could feel the tears welling up . . . I knew she wasn't going to be there when I came on duty the next day.'

In another case, a patient died suddenly of a heart attack while in hospital, and a nurse reported: 'It was difficult because we tried to resuscitate her and to no avail, so then you think you've failed, you've got that sense of failure as well. You've also got the shock of it happening and the business of having to inform the relative.'

A hospice nurse described a patient with whom she identified, who was admitted and had a paracentesis (removal of fluid from a cavity in the body) and was expected to go home, but the following day she died.

> I felt I'd let her down because, when she had the paracentesis, I'd gone off and I said, 'I'll see you tomorrow and this time next week you'll be going out.' And when I came on the next day she was critical . . . I don't know, whether I put so much effort into it or whether I felt kicked in the teeth because she was dying or we'd let her down or would she have been better without the paracentesis? I couldn't explain to anybody how upset I felt. And for a while, when anybody came in with a paracentesis, I got the heebie-jeebies.

From the above experiences it would seem that identification processes and sudden death may make feeling that you have let a patient down more likely.

In some situations the reactions of professional helpers may be similar to those of patients and relatives. A social worker described a young family she was working with: a man had been diagnosed with lung cancer and inoperable brain secondaries 3 weeks previously. He was told that he had about 2 months to live, if that. They had two boys aged 9 and 7 and his wife had just had twins. This worker's reaction was to blame God: 'I think, "How on earth can you do this?" I have great difficulty, like families do, finding a reason. When they say, "Why?" I'm thinking, "Well, I'm asking why as well!" It just seems so senseless, so awful, that that should happen.'

This is similar to the response of a teacher interviewed by one of the authors. When talking to her young class following the death of one of their fellow pupils, she found it hard to answer questions about why God had allowed him to die. The same questions had occurred to her.

Finally in this section, it is important to remind ourselves of the other side of the coin: that in working with dying people it is possible to be affected in a positive way. One hospice worker talked of finding it humbling to see people show such courage in the face of horrible disease. 'It's a tremendous privilege to know some of these patients.'

The notion of caring for a dying person being a 'gift' is alluded to by Lee (1995). A woman who looked after her mother at home during her terminal illness talked of being given something and of it being a very precious thing to be allowed to look after her. Similarly, a nurse interviewed by one of the authors talked in terms of a patient's disease, suffering and death being a gift to the nurse, which could act as a catalyst for personal growth. For this to happen there has to be a relationship between patient and nurse that is not based on fear and distancing.

In this section we have illustrated some of the ways professional helpers can be affected in their work with dying people. Clearly some of these reactions can be associated with high levels of distress and point to the need for emotional support (Chapter 16).

To summarize, in this chapter we have described some of the theoretical attempts to understand the process of dying and highlighted the importance of not making assumptions about what individual dying patients may be thinking or feeling. We have also addressed some of the factors that can affect relatives (such as anticipatory grief) and professional helpers (such as feeling they have let the patient down). Broader issues of grief and caring for the dying person will be discussed in the next chapter.

Issues of grief and caring for the dying person

9

Being truly present means that the caregiver is with the person physically, emotionally and spiritually, focusing his or her attention on the present time, in the present place, with the present person.

Samarel, 1995

These patients were being 'held back' by something still undone. These unresolved issues usually were related to a need for reconciliation – to finish unfinished business.

Callanan and Kelley, 1992

Moving a dying patient is usually more distressing than leaving him where he is because it makes other patients question what death is like and think, 'It must be dreadful if we are never allowed to see it.'

Dame Cicely Saunders, quoted by Sadler, 1992

Caring well for a dying person raises many issues, not just about death but also about life, the way it is lived and what it means to be one human being in relation to another. It also poses the question of time: do we have time to be alongside someone who is dying and share in the grief? As pointed out in Chapter 6, it is also important to say, 'I am going to die,' to ourselves before working with the dying, otherwise our own unsaid fears and anxieties may get in the way.

In this chapter we address the question of what dying people need, including help with completing unfinished business; also how we respond to death, for example in relation to other patients, and ways of comforting and connecting with the dying.

WHAT DO DYING PEOPLE MOST NEED?

The responses of two nurses to this question included:

- somebody with them, somebody sometimes just to sit beside them;
- comfort, somebody touching them, somebody holding their hand;

- somebody to talk to;
- somebody who cares about them.

These comments emphasize the importance of communication and caring. Grollman (1995) talks of the value of having someone who cares about you in relation to bereavement but his comments apply equally to someone who is dying:

A person who will share with you
the agony of your grief
so that on your sorrowing path
you do not walk alone.

There may be all sorts of reasons why it is difficult to be alongside someone who is dying. Some of these were discussed in Chapter 2 and include being under a high level of stress and feeling undervalued. In such circumstances it may be difficult to muster up any spare 'emotional energy'. Quoist (1965) uses an analogy to describe how we might not have time for others because we are too 'filled up'. If you have been waiting for a bus for some time and then it passes you by all filled up, you may get annoyed, especially if it happens often. Similarly, some people may always be filled up with themselves and so pass by others. Yet, as Quoist (1965) puts it in addressing the individual: 'No one else will stop at this particular place and at this particular time. Only you can pick up this person here and now.'

An example of this situation is the professional helper who talked about a conversation she had with her father, who had cancer:

I took him to all his appointments. I remember quite well when he was really poorly with radiotherapy and he said, 'I can't see the point in going on.' We just didn't mention the word cancer but at that moment he really did give me the perfect opening for discussion . . . I shut the door on him, I changed the subject and he never spoke again about his illness.

A hospice nurse, talking about learning from patients, had received positive feedback about being a good listener. However, the comment had also been made to her, 'You're always in a rush,' and her reaction to this was: 'It brings you up with a jolt because you're not fulfilling your role if you're always in a rush.'

The issue of the relationship between our own preoccupations and feelings and our ability to give to others is discussed by Larson (1993). For example, he discusses how lack of time hinders helping by reference to the 'Good Samaritan' experiments of Darley and Batson (1973). Theology students were asked to walk across campus to give a talk on the parable of the Good Samaritan. They came across a slumped 'victim' on their way across campus. In this experiment some students were told to hurry and others to walk leisurely. Some 63% of the students who were not hurrying offered help and only 10% of those who were hurrying provided help. In contrast to the latter situation, when we are feeling good, for example after receiving positive feedback or a thank you, our assessment of how much we can afford to give to others is altered. We are more likely to share this good feeling with those less fortunate and be less concerned about the returns from our giving.

Wright (1988) asked the question, 'What would I most need if I was terminally ill?' and described four areas:

- to be helped to know very gently that I am dying and to be enabled to face my dying properly; this would include making necessary arrangements and saying thank you and goodbye (this issue will be discussed in Chapter 11);
- to know that I will be supported to the end and never abandoned; that I will be helped to fulfil the hope that I am going to live until the moment I die;
- somebody who will listen to me, for example if there is something I am ashamed of, something I want to 'get rid of' or offload;
- somebody who will share in my helplessness.

To summarize these observations: dying people first of all need others who are not too full of their own difficulties – someone who is able to be with and alongside them and share in their helplessness; and someone who will listen at the right time. For some professional helpers who are used to doing things for people, this element of 'being with' people may not come easily.

FACILITATING THE COMPLETION OF UNFINISHED BUSINESS

The term 'unfinished business' refers to unresolved difficulties or regrets that may interfere with being at peace. Examples include estrangement within the family and selfish things we have done. Buckman (1996b) describes how life-threatening illness 'telescopes the future': in other words, our time scale is reduced, so that anxiety or guilt about unfinished business may suddenly be magnified. This may apply particularly to secrets. Lee (1995) gives some examples, including having a criminal record, having had a baby who was 'given away' for adoption, being a secret homosexual and one's financial affairs being in a mess. A current love affair while still in a relationship with one's spouse can be a particularly distressing form of unfinished business. Parkes et al. (1996) also discuss how secrets can cause difficulties for, for example, lesbians and gay men, whose relationships may be known only to a few people. This may result in them mourning alone and the impact of their loss going unrecognized.

Ward (1993) includes saying goodbye under the heading of dealing with unfinished business. However, this seems to be inappropriate except in particular circumstances, for example when saying goodbye involves expressing feelings that have formerly remained hidden.

A general nurse on an oncology ward worked with a man who had terminal cancer. He had not had contact with his son for several years, following a family argument. One night the nurse sat with this man as he talked about his regrets over the stupid family argument and the nasty things they'd said to each other. He hadn't got in touch with his son for fear of being rejected. The nurse had commented, 'Well you never know, you could die never knowing.' This patient wrote a letter to his son and got a reply. However, the nurse then left the ward so was unaware as to whether the two actually met.

In another case, a son had not seen his father for 8 or 9 years until he visited his dying father in a hospice. The nurse had to act as a go-between when the son just turned up one day. She had to ask the patient if he would see his son, then leave them once they had started communicating. The patient died a few days later.

Sometimes a dying person may be tempted to write a letter or record a tape that could leave unfinished business for the recipient. In this scenario, one social worker reported that she would try to get the two people together. She would act as a catalyst and break the ice to help them start communicating, then take a back seat when no longer needed.

Unfinished business may sometimes be recent and related to the process of care rather than to distant unresolved difficulties. This can apply when patients feel angry about being 'dumped' in hospital or a hospice and the relatives may feel guilty that they have let the patient down. Helping people to express their feelings and pointing out the value of shared care can be useful in this situation. Also, on a day-to-day basis a relative may have regrets after a particular visit. One relative telephoned a hospice after an evening visit, 'When I came in, my mother shouted at me and I shouted back ... I wouldn't want ...' In response, the nurse encouraged the relative to come back to the hospice that evening.

In this kind of situation the role of the professional helper can involve listening, reflecting, negotiating, ice-breaking and generally helping to facilitate meaningful communication between patients and relatives. It may include helping to prevent new unfinished business from arising as well as reconciling past difficulties.

Callanan and Kelley (1992) describe how dying people may give messages concerning the need for reconciliation and that these messages need to be interpreted. An example is a dying woman whose father-in-law couldn't cope with the prospect of her death and so didn't visit. This woman, fairly close to death, was heard to say repeatedly, 'We must go to the park.' Her husband realized that this referred to when she used to often go to the park with his father and the children. Her father-in-law was brought to her and there was reconciliation before her death that evening. Sometimes the message may indicate a need for forgiveness as in the case of the war veteran who had served in Vietnam. His confused speech included words such as, 'villages', 'babies', 'napalm', 'burning' and 'I did it.' It wasn't until a chaplain visited that his anguished crying slowly stopped and he died a few hours later.

In a third example, Callanan and Kelley (1992) describe a dying woman who lived with a man she loved but could not marry him because her ex-husband would not agree to a divorce. When enough time had elapsed legally for her to get a divorce she had developed cancer and her ex-husband threatened to declare her mentally incompetent because of the extent of her illness. She was heard to often be saying the word 'rings' and this message was interpreted as an indication of her desperate wish to be married. A chaplain performed a ceremony to bless their loving relationship and her husband put a ring on her thin finger, even though they could not legally marry. That night was their first peaceful one in 3 weeks and she died the next morning.

These observations indicate that what is actually needed to complete unfinished business may not always be obvious and that professional helpers need to work with relatives to interpret the messages. This applies particularly to patients who are near to death, whose speech may not be easily understood.

Ideally, of course, unfinished business should be addressed well before one's last days or hours of life. Professional helpers could ask dying people questions such as:

- 'People sometimes bottle up their thoughts and feelings and it can be helpful to talk about them. I wonder if you have any thoughts or feelings you would like to talk about?'
- 'Are there any important things you would like to talk about, either today or at some other time?'
- 'Is there anyone special you would like to visit you?'

Another approach is to encourage people to carry out a life review, i.e. to talk about what they are proud of and what has been a disappointment to them (see, for instance, Haight, 1988; Garland, 1994). Both these approaches, if carried out in the context of a trusting relationship, are likely to uncover the need to complete any unfinished business.

SAYING GOODBYE AND 'FUTURE PRESENCE'

If one is prepared for death and has come to terms with it in the sense of reaching a level of acceptance, then saying goodbye is likely to be easier. Lee (1995) describes the activities of a woman 2 weeks before she died. These included deciding together with her daughter-in-law who should have her jewellery, discussing the afterlife with a grandson and planning her funeral. She also reviewed her life with her daughter-in-law and her two sisters and their husbands. All these actions can be viewed as part of the process of saying goodbye.

Action that aims to maintain one's presence at significant times in the future may be taken because of a feeling that one cannot properly say goodbye, and to help relatives who are left behind. This seems to apply particularly when a parent with young children is dying. A young woman who was dying had three children aged 5, 7 and 10 years and she wrote letters to all of them, with the help of a nurse who sat with her and assisted with spelling. The letters included one for when the children got married. She also wrote that she would like the first grand-child to be called after her and wondered aloud with the nurse whether this was selfish. The nurse commented that it wasn't really selfish and was able to bring an element of humour to the situation by pointing out that it would be a silly name to call a boy.

Another way of viewing this projecting of oneself into the future is that it is a compensation for 'loss of oughts' (Chapter 4). In the example just quoted, the loss was not seeing one's children grow up and not being there at significant times in their lives.

If what one is going to leave for the future is discussed with or prepared jointly with those who will be left behind, this may assist with the process of saying goodbye. A 'memory store' could include letters, audio or video tapes, personal objects or keepsakes that have shared personal significance for the dying person and his/her relatives.

Leaving a written or recorded message may also be helpful if dying people find it difficult to express their feelings verbally face to face. (As pointed out earlier in this chapter, though, this would not be appropriate if the message left the recipient with unfinished business.) The message might include valued shared memories and expressions of love.

ENABLING THE GRIEF OF OTHER PATIENTS

> Why do we screen them off? You screen them off and then there's this very secretive thing. You screen every patient off while the porters come and collect the body and then you leave the curtains round. Every patient on that ward knows there's been a death but it's never spoken about.

This is a nurse's description of procedures on her ward when a patient's body is removed. There is a clear symbolism in the act of drawing curtains round patients' beds and 'protecting' them from the sight of death. Rational arguments for this might include the observation that the process of removing the body is not very dignified. However, presumably the prime reason for screening off is based on a notion that if other patients were to see the dead patient being taken out it would be too upsetting for them. But what about their private thoughts? These might include:

- 'I wonder how she died?'
- 'I've not had a chance to pay my last respects.'
- 'She had similar problems to me; am I going to die? Will I die like that?'

There is some evidence to suggest that not protecting other patients from death can be helpful. Johnston *et al.* (1992) carried out a study with 11 patients in a hospice setting who had shared a small ward with a patient who had died. Their reactions were compared with those of nine other patients who had not observed the death of another patient. Those who had witnessed a death were less depressed and rated the death of another patient as significantly more comforting than distressing. Also, more patients said it would be worse for them if a dying patient were moved out of their ward area. It seems that reassurance was being provided by seeing that people can die peacefully. Although a small-scale study, it highlights the importance of not making assumptions about how other patients may be affected by a death.

Abdel-Fattah *et al.* (1992) make some useful suggestions for talking to other patients, including using phrases like 'has died' rather than euphemisms like 'was taken from us' and allowing them to ask questions – 'I wondered if you wanted to ask me any questions?' If a patient dies an unusually distressing death it may be helpful to communicate the message: 'The way that this disease affected that patient was unusual.' Issues about not breaking confidentiality need to be kept in mind.

When another patient had made friends with the patient who died, the grief may be greater, so it is probably even more important to be open. Good practice here is illustrated in the following example from a hospice worker: 'Two men here recently made a good friend of each other and one died. I went to say I was sorry and do you want to talk about it? How has it affected you and what do you think?' This approach gives patients the opportunity to express their feelings and to ask questions like 'Is that how it will be for me?'

There are a number of ways in which patients could be helped to acknowledge the death of a fellow patient. If they had made friends, they may wish to write to the relatives, send flowers or, state of health permitting, attend the funeral. Another possibility is to have a short service on the ward to coincide with the time of the actual funeral (Chapter 10). In a hospice setting where there are regular services in the chapel, a candle may be lit and a remembrance period included in the service. Another idea is to have a remembrance book. Other patients, particularly those who had become friends, may wish to see the body when laid out and say their goodbyes. This may need to be checked out with any relatives first to make sure that they have no objections.

Although it would not be deemed as appropriate in Western culture, Lee (1995) describes an experience that is in stark contrast to the 'screening off' described at the beginning of this section. A student doctor was attempting cardiac massage on a woman in a maternity ward in Kenya. The patient's mother leant across her dead daughter and pushed the doctor away. Then she stood up and with one arm raised above her head, began to sing a hymn. All the other patients on the ward stood by their beds with faces turned to the dead woman and sang with her mother. Even though this approach could not be applied literally in our culture, it could serve as a useful image to keep in mind when exploring ways of helping other patients to acknowledge a patient's death. It is an image that symbolizes facing and acknowledging death rather than hiding it.

'COMFORTING' COMMUNICATION

Bottorff *et al.* (1995) carried out a study involving eight inpatients with cancer and 32 nurses. Several hundred hours of video-tape data were collected and analysed and various comforting interactions were described. These included:

GENTLE HUMOUR

Humorous statements were made in connection with patients, their illness or the nurses themselves and nurses sometimes used gentle forms of teasing. Social touch was sometimes used with humour to convey the message that the nurse was not really serious. Also, it was noted that nurses used gentle humour as a means of helping patients to relax.

PROVIDING INFORMATION

Information was provided on topics such as the patient's illness and treatment, the hospital environment and staff. Giving realistic expectations about a patient's illness or care appeared to have the potential to reduce anxieties. Various techniques were used by nurses to ensure that patients understood and assimilated information, including minimizing jargon, repeating key ideas, using gestures for emphasis, clear articulation and checking, either verbally or by picking up non-verbal cues (from facial expression), that the patients had understood.

EMOTIONALLY SUPPORTIVE STATEMENTS

Communicating emotional support partly involved using a basic coun-selling approach, for instance reflecting back patients' concerns (Chapter 14). It also included providing encouragement and commiserating. Making such emotionally supportive statements created an atmosphere of acceptance that seemed to help patients feel free to discuss their experiences and feelings.

INVOLVEMENT IN CARE

Patients were actively encouraged to participate in decisions about their care, thereby introducing an element of control for them. For example, nurses asked specific questions such as 'Would you like to bathe now or later in the day?' and 'Where do you want your subcutaneous site this time?' They also asked more general open-ended questions such as 'What else can I do for you?'

SOCIAL EXCHANGE

Informal friendly conversation about everyday things was another comforting strategy that enabled patients to step out of their sick role for a while. It served, for example, to lighten the atmosphere and keep patients in touch with the outside world and it was observed that patients often responded positively to such exchanges.

INCREASING PROXIMITY AND TOUCH

Nurses increased their proximity, for example by standing close to or sitting on the patient's bed. They encouraged patients to talk by providing feedback such as nodding or saying 'Go on'. Increasing prox-imity was a way for nurses to indicate their willingness to be close and share patients' experiences, especially if the patient was distressed.

Two types of touch were observed: comforting and connecting. Comforting touch was used to reassure or calm patients and included stroking their arms, backs or legs and covering or holding their hands. Connecting touch was used by nurses to show their interest in patients or to reassure them when leaving the room. An example was observed after a long, late-night discussion with a patient who couldn't sleep; the nurse lightly touched the patient's hand as she left to get an analgesic for him.

Some of these comforting interactions are similar to the elements of what Nichols (1993) describes as psychological care. This includes infor-mational/educational care, emotional care, basic counselling and advo-cacy (representing the needs of the patient).

The interesting and positive aspect of the above study by Bottorff *et al.* (1995) is that the various comforting interactions took place during the normal day-to-day contact between patients and nurses. This partly addresses the question raised at the beginning of this chapter – do we have time to be alongside someone who is dying?

Autton (1996) describes the use of touch as a way of expressing 'alongsideness' without appearing to patronize: 'A caring touch demonstrates empathy and is one way of "giving permission" to patients and relatives to reveal their anxieties and distress.'

Older (1982) also observed that actually touching people during an examination (as opposed to just using medical instruments) often leads to them opening up and telling you things they wouldn't otherwise have said. One general nurse reported how patients often talked about things that were important to them while she was doing shoulder or back massage and that this was less likely, for example, if she was doing hand massage. During massage patients may feel that they are very special to the nurse and trust may be built up. In this context, talking more freely about important concerns when there is no eye contact may be possible because patients do not have to be concerned about non-verbal signals, either those they may be conveying or those that the nurse may transmit from facial expression.

Another interesting example of what can facilitate important discussion is provided by an experience of Colin Murray-Parkes (Parkes *et al.*, 1996). He asked a patient who had complained of pain in the night what she had wanted from the night staff. She replied, 'a cup of tea,' because she knew that the nurse would sit and talk to her while she drank it. It transpired that she wanted to talk about the fact that she had cancer and her fears about it.

Teaching a relative to do, for example, a simple hand or foot massage can also enhance communication between relative and patient. The use of aromatherapy can also facilitate communication; one nurse has found that lavender can trigger off reminiscing in older patients, which could in turn help with the process of life review mentioned earlier in this chapter. Shenton (1996) quotes the example of a terminally ill, blind man who reported feeling 'cared for' when receiving hand massage with oils from an aromatherapist. He had no living friends or relatives and the therapy appeared to reduce his sense of isolation.

Although it may be difficult to describe and 'pin down' as a skill, some nurses may develop a high level of empathy, which enables them to tune in to a patient's feelings. This is illustrated by the following comments of a nurse whose work included care of dying patients:

> We've got a lady at the moment who's dying and people say that she's completely accepting it because she talks about it to her family. But she hasn't, she lies on her bed and I can hear her weeping

and I think she thinks it isn't going to happen. Now she's getting more symptoms and she's really frightened. You can see it in her eyes and you can feel it as you talk to her.

If you sit close enough, they'll often need to touch, even those who haven't wanted it before suddenly seem to need to touch. They feel isolated and alone and I can feel those feelings.

Although paying attention to non-verbal cues is clearly important in these examples, such empathy is probably only likely to develop when the helper is able to be fully attentive to and 'present' with patients during any interactions with them. This requires helpers to temporarily shelve any hassles or difficulties they may be experiencing.

To recap, important factors that enable getting alongside dying people include the following:

- saying to ourselves, 'I am going to die,' so that fears about our own mortality don't get in the way;
- being supported so that our own stresses don't get in the way;
- feeling valued so that we can in turn value the dying;
- using a range of 'comforting' strategies;
- responding at the time a patient chooses to open up to us by listening;
- conveying the message that we have time by not always being in a rush;
- facilitating the completion of unfinished business;
- facilitating saying goodbye and any preparation for 'future presence';
- enabling other patients who are dying to face grief when a patient dies.

The reader will probably have noticed that these factors are a mixture of knowledge, social and other skills, a willingness to consider personal matters, and organizational issues. The latter can help to create the right psychological/social environment and atmosphere by valuing and supporting helpers and not putting them under too much pressure.

In this chapter we have considered what dying people need, including help with issues they may need to resolve, in order to have a peaceful death. Ways of connecting with and getting alongside patients and approaches to helping them to face death, rather than protecting them from it, have also been explored. All these approaches, which do not rely on lengthy counselling sessions, should be practically possible and it is hoped that the reader will have been assisted in his or her efforts to care well for dying people.

Religious, spiritual and cultural needs 10

It is one of the developmental tasks of the maturing psyche to come to terms with death.

Stedeford, 1984

It is essential to consider what spiritual care each patient may need, and to make it available to him, in response to his own unique need.

Pass, 1989

Spiritual pain, then, is not so much 'a problem to be solved', as 'a question to be lived'.

Elsdon, 1995

Hunkin (1987) has said that 'the twentieth century has been essentially the age of the half believer'. In Hunkin's view, people today still retain a latent religious belief system but are confused by modern theology.

While formal religion for much of the Western world is at its lowest ebb, religion is not itself completely moribund. There are still a minority of people who would claim to be devout followers of their particular faith. Others who would only admit to a nominal interest in religion might, at moments of crisis, find comfort in religious practices.

There are many people today who would profess to no active participation in religion. Some, indeed, would claim to be atheists, but would nevertheless acknowledge a spiritual element to their lives. They would distinguish this belief from religion, or religious belief.

Sir Ludovic Kennedy in a *Sunday Times Magazine* article (5th November 1995) writes, 'I think it's a mistake to confuse spiritualism with faith. There is spirituality in nature, in emotional relationships, in poetry. Whenever I see the vastness of the ocean or the sky at night, I feel part of it. But that doesn't make me believe that there is a God.'

At its best, religion is an expression of a deep spirituality. In theistic religions, this finds expression in a desire for a personal relationship with the deity. In non-theistic religions it expresses itself in a seeking of a oneness with the universe. For those who profess to have no religion, spirituality may involve an awareness of another dimension to life, of meaning and purpose outside of the material; or simply a questioning of these things in non-religious terms. Peberdy (1993) writes, 'Perhaps it may help to see spirituality as search for meaning and religion as a particular expression of that.' As one woman who practised no religion said to one of the authors, 'When I see people around me dying, and I've always been ill, I wonder what I was put on this earth for? What was I supposed to do?'

There are yet others for whom religion is diffuse and unconsidered. It finds expression in deeply felt cultural rituals that may have no foundation in formal theology. Some might disparagingly refer to such beliefs as 'folk religion' or 'superstition'. However the reader views it or, indeed, views any religious practice, the rituals often express very deeply held beliefs. It is important that the validity of these beliefs be acknowledged for the individual and, wherever possible, their expression facilitated.

These three strands, then, of religion, spirituality and cultural need are often confused. But, as Ross (1994a) in her doctoral study found, nurses had 'a propensity to view spiritual needs in religious terms'.

It is our intention in this chapter to disentangle some of the threads. This will include outlining some of the important spiritual, religious and cultural needs and giving some ideas to help carers facilitate the meeting of some of these needs. We will be looking at these issues under the following headings.

- What is the role of religion?
- How does spirituality differ from religion?
- The dying patient and some rites of passage.
- What is the role of cultural and ritual practice?
- Religious needs and the role of the chaplain.
- How can we help to facilitate the meeting of spiritual needs?

WHAT IS THE ROLE OF RELIGION?

Hospice staff we interviewed felt that not all religious people, even deeply religious people, find that their religion is a help to them when they or their relatives are terminally ill. For some the nature of their religious beliefs brings fear and anxiety rather than comfort. As a senior hospice nurse said in an interview, 'Sometimes the patients who are the more religious are the more frightened at the end,' or, as Ross (1997) writes, 'For many people, however, the experiences of hospitalization, illness and – in particular – terminal illness may precipitate spiritual distress. These experiences may cause some individuals to lose control for the first time in their lives.'

For many, however, religion brings a special comfort and eases their death, or the grief of relatives when someone close to them dies. It can also prove helpful to some people who appear not to be religious. As a hospice counsellor remarked, 'The other thing I've experienced is that people who have no faith can suddenly become very religious, and want all the religious trappings, and want to talk in very over-religious terms.'

This book is not intended to be a theological treatise, so for our purposes we will define religion simply as, firstly, a systematized belief system that seeks to make sense of the world, secondly as the expression of that belief in ritual, thirdly as the observance of moral codes and finally as the making sense of the universe in a belief system that seeks to account for the way that things are. This is sometimes expressed within theistic faiths in a personal relationship with the deity, and involves what are considered by their followers to be means of communication with the deity. This communication may include prayer, the reading of sacred books or meditation.

For those who are practising members of a religion their faith has two important dimensions for us to consider. It involves a relationship with the deity (or a spiritual discipline) that needs to be maintained. Often this takes the form of rituals or formalized procedures. The Muslim, for instance, needs, wherever possible, to pray five times a day facing in the direction of Mecca. It is helpful if staff are aware of these needs and can facilitate meeting them.

The second dimension is that of belonging to a group of fellow believers, 'the community of faith'. Some of the practices of the various religions serve the function of reinforcing that sense of belonging. In the majority of Christian denominations, the Eucharist serves both as a means of bonding with God and as something that binds the people of God together. (See Religious needs and the role of the chaplain, below.) It is essentially a corporate activity. It serves to remind individuals, even if they are alone with their pastor in taking communion, that they are sharing in a 'family meal' with their fellow Christians.

If patients are denied these opportunities to practise their religion, then the sense of alienation and fear that may well be present for a number of those who are dying will increase.

Firth (1993) writes, 'Ignorance and lack of sensitivity on the part of medical or social work personnel about the religious beliefs and cultural outlook of patients can make an already frightening situation worse, particularly in hospital, where language may be an additional barrier.'

In addition many religions have spiritual practices that have to do with the end of life. These have come to be known collectively as 'rites of passage'. They are ritual practices that are designed to ease the patient's passing out of this life. The phrase 'the last rites' does not simply apply to those Catholic wings of the Church that administer extreme unction – what is now referred to as 'anointing the sick' (see Hollins, 1989) – but also to many other rites in the Christian churches, and in other religions too. The failure to administer these rites may make for considerable dis-ease in terminally ill people. Conversely, their administration may be extremely helpful in bringing peace and calm.

Whatever our personal views of religion, or if the religious beliefs of patients are different from our own, it is the responsibility of all who have care for the dying to help to ensure that those needs are met.

HOW DOES SPIRITUALITY DIFFER FROM RELIGION?

We have already skirted round this issue, but it is important to make a clear distinction between religion and spirituality. Religion at its worst is a set of ritual practices devoid of meaning, an unconsidered habit. At its best, it is the expression of a deeply felt spirituality that finds meaning in the beliefs and activities of the religion that is espoused.

We are faced with a difficulty when seeking to define spirituality because by its very nature spirituality is concerned with our awareness of the transcendent, that which is beyond ourselves. Spirituality is easier to perceive than it is to explain.

The word spirituality is used in two related but distinct senses. We use it to describe that experience of awe, of wonder and delight that many experience when listening to great music, viewing a painting or responding to some new appreciation of nature. When we are moved by these things, we may describe the experience we have as spiritual. This is the aspect of spirituality that Sir Ludovic Kennedy was describing earlier. Although Charles Wesley, in his hymn 'Love Divine, All Loves Excelling', was writing about a religious experience when he penned the line 'Lost in wonder, love and praise', his description would equally fit any deeply meaningful spiritual experience.

We also use the word 'spirituality' to denote our search for the ultimate meanings of life. Ross (1994a) states that many authors 'regard the need for meaning as a universal trait that is essential to life itself'. It is our spiritual understanding of the world and of our place in it, of the duration and meaning of existence, that gives shape to the way that we are in the world. It helps define our morals and our attitudes to all around us.

Spirituality has been defined as 'a way of being and experiencing that comes about through awareness of a transcendent dimension and that is characterized by certain identifiable values in regard to self, others, nature, life, and whatever one considers to be the Ultimate' (Elkins, *et al.*, 1988). Alternatively, Dickenson and Johnson (1993) write, 'Perhaps it may help to see spirituality as a search for meaning and religion as a particular expression of that (one that usually involves God-language).'

Cornette (1997) reports on research done by LUCAS where a questionnaire was sent out to 841 palliative health workers from the Flemish-speaking area of Belgium. A total of 429 replies were received; 90.2% agreed with definitions of religion and spirituality formulated by the LUCAS team. These definitions are:

- **spirituality**: concerning that dynamic within each human being to situate oneself in a horizon that gives meaning to different life experiences;
- **religion**: concerning that particular form of spirituality that places human beings in relation to (a) God.

This appears to us to be a useful definition of spirituality but the definition of religion fails to encompass the Buddhists and others who would acknowledge no belief in a God or gods.

For some, ideas of spirituality are confined to formal religion. However, as we have seen from the above, this is a restricted view. In the course of an interview a hospice counsellor said, 'I think the only thing I would add is that to be aware that people have spiritual needs. I think too often we talk about being religious and we dismiss the spiritual.'

Elsdon (1995) makes the point that 'Spiritual needs are distinct from religious needs, and this is an area where a great deal of misunderstanding can occur: the words "spiritual" and "religious" are often used synonymously, although they are separate – if related – dimensions.'

Many people therefore dismiss the idea of the spiritual because in their minds it is synonymous with religion. Not considering themselves to be religious, they therefore assume that they are not spiritual either. This feeling is compounded by the way in which spirituality tends to be spoken of in religious terms. One nurse, relating how a hospital chaplain discussed in a pilot workshop the concept of spiritual needs, said that 'he'd got his own terminology'. The result of this was that this nurse, who was a cofacilitator, felt that they had 'lost the whole thing' and that she would want to use a different set of words. She would use language that would communicate spirituality without couching it in religious terms. She also found in the course of her work that many of the colleagues she worked with had 'a spiritual aspect to them that they did not recognize'.

As mentioned in Chapter 8, Maslow (1987) put forward the idea that we all have a hierarchy of needs. At the base of what he describes as a pyramid are our physiological needs. When those needs are met, the next most paramount are the needs of safety and security, then love and belonging, followed by self-esteem and finally, at the apex, self-actualization.

Sheila Cassidy, in a seminar with health-care chaplains attended by one of the authors, modified this pyramid by placing spiritual need at the apex in the place of self-actualization. The point that she was making was that all other needs have to be met before the patient is able to take account of his or her spiritual needs. While this is undoubtedly true, for some dying patients who realize that death is approaching it may be that lesser needs cease to be so important. There could be an increasing emphasis on spiritual needs.

Focusing on spiritual needs may lead to some important changes for the person. Du Boulay (1984), writing on the work of Cicely Saunders, records a conversation a patient had with a staff nurse. 'I feel I am going to find, if I have the time, another way of life, not dramatic, perhaps not even very different, but something that will be the best in my life.'

A nurse who works on an elderly care ward illustrated this when she described her experience of nursing someone with multiple sclerosis whom she spoke of as 'severely diseased, but whole'.

THE DYING PATIENT AND SOME RITES OF PASSAGE

In this section we will be looking at cultural and religious practice for patients who are dying and their relatives. In the next section we will consider those rituals that have to do with the preparation of the body for burial.

Dying is a physical process but it also has psychological and spiritual dimensions. In this section we will deal with the psychological and spiritual, specifically as they relate to cultural and ritual practice.

Dying can be a frightening experience. It can also be very lonely. Anything that eases the fear, or brings comfort to the dying patient, is to be welcomed. Because in dying we can become alienated from the living, it is important as far as possible to maintain those things that give stability and security to the patient. Diet, for instance, is often a very important cultural component of the lives of many people whose ethnic origin is in the East. Serving standard English food to someone who relates culturally to India, for instance, could add a further sense of alienation to them. Washing in running water for Muslims, the wearing of sacred emblems for the Sikhs and, for some Christians, the practice of daily Bible reading are important aids towards maintaining spiritual equilibrium at a time when they may be experiencing spiritual and emotional disorientation. Those who care for the dying should be aware of this and seek to provide the relevant practical help wherever possible.

In addition, certain rites of passage may be of help to some people – as for instance the anointing with oil referred to earlier, or a religious or cultural memento. Clark and Jacinta (1995) write, 'For some a religious memento is important and for some Roman Catholic families a crucifix or rosary may be placed in the hands of a dead person.' In terms of objects or rituals that bring comfort, we should remember that something as mundane as an evening glass of whisky for someone who has followed the pattern of a daily tipple for many years may be equally helpful. If we cannot provide what is needed, then perhaps a chaplain may be able to help.

When the patient has died, the needs of his or her relatives become paramount. However it can also be important for the patient to know that the correct ritual will be performed after he or she has died.

It might be helpful to consider a cultural ritual that we often take for granted. Where there are no religious strictures regarding last offices, nurses tend to 'lay out' patients according to a standard pattern. To what extent do tasks performed in last offices have practical justification, and how much is culturally determined? For instance, why do we tend to dress the body in a shroud rather than in the patient's clothes? Why do we close the eyes and ensure that the mouth is closed? Clark and Jacinta (1995) point out that last offices play an important role in affording dignity to the deceased. 'Last offices have always been recognized as the final service offered as a mark of respect to the dead person before burial or cremation.'

Each of the major religions have their own requirements with respect to last offices and the reader is encouraged to read, for example, Clark and Jacinta (1995), Neuberger (1987), Dickenson and Johnson (1993) for a fuller picture of the needs of different cultures with respect to last offices.

WHAT IS THE ROLE OF CULTURAL AND RITUAL PRACTICE?

Firth (1993) says that 'Religious and cultural rituals invest death with meaning from religious, psychological and social perspectives.' This is illustrated in more specific terms by Arnold Van Gennep, who first coined the term 'rites of passage'. He said that these rituals had three functions; separation, transition and incorporation. There has to be, first, a group acknowledgement that death has actually occurred. It needs to be recognized that the dead person's status in the group has changed, as in the styles 'Mr John Smith (deceased)' or 'the late Joan Green'. Next, there needs to be a time allowed for the implications of this loss and separation to set in. Finally, the group needs to affirm cohesiveness in spite of the loss of one of its members.

So in England, when someone dies, the body is ritually prepared for burial (last offices). The body is then placed in a coffin. This is often left open for relatives to view the body in the funeral parlour. This is the first stage, separation. The funeral then marks the second stage, that of transition. The third phase, incorporation, is seen in the funeral tea, where members of the family and close friends gather to affirm again the unity of the group.

Rituals also have another function, that of validating and affirming a change from one state of being into another. Those changes affect our role in society; they bring with them the authority of the state or community. So in a wedding ceremony, for instance, the officially sanctioned registrar or minister performs this role, as does the one who directs at any rite of passage for the dying person and his or her relatives.

RELIGIOUS/SPIRITUAL NEEDS AND THE ROLE OF THE CHAPLAIN

What is the role of the chaplain? In the authors' experience there is more than a little confusion as to the chaplain's task in the hospital. McGregor (1990) writes, 'In both acute and long stay wards, chaplaincy is most acceptable and effective when integrated into a programme of treatment and care shared with other health-service professionals.' Some chaplains may experience this situation, especially if they are full-time. The reality for part-time chaplains, however, is often very different. The chaplain's role varies not only from hospital to hospital but even from one ward to another within the same hospital.

In one ward the chaplain may find that he or she is recognized as a valuable part of the therapeutic team while in another the chaplain is considered to be just another visitor. This latter situation is epitomized by one incident, experienced by one of the authors, where he was in deep conversation with a patient only to be interrupted while a nurse took a blood pressure. (There was no hint that the timing of this procedure was critical.)

The chaplain's role is to provide the link between the hospital and the community of faith, which is often perceived to be external to the hospital walls. Often the patient feels cut off from his or her spiritual, cultural, and religious roots in what can sometimes feel like an alien environment.

In order to form the bridge between the community outside the hospital and the environment within, the chaplain seeks to bring the services of the Church to the patient, administering communion, baptism or other service as required. In certain long-stay wards in psychiatric hospitals a simple memorial service is sometimes conducted on the ward for patients who cannot attend a partner's funeral, or for other patients when a resident dies. Often this service is timed to coincide with the actual funeral and uses the same readings and prayers. Chaplains also function on behalf of patients as a link with leaders of other faiths, should a visit be requested.

As well as seeking to help meet the spiritual needs of patients of all faiths and none, the chaplains have a role too in seeking to help the patient's relatives, and the chaplain is also there for the spiritual needs of the staff.

On long-stay wards, chaplains often get to know the patients well and may therefore be aware of their spiritual needs. Very rarely, though, will chaplains know patients as well as do the nurses, who care for them over a much longer time span and who are also involved with those patients in a much more intimate way. Elsdon (1995) writes, 'Nurses spend more time with terminally ill patients than most; they are often the ones to whom a patient will turn in spiritual distress, and are therefore in an excellent position to help a person with spiritual pain.' These observations illustrate the potential value of team work.

In acute areas, patients may not even be aware of the existence of the chaplain, or the chaplain of them (except as a name on the bed state list). This inevitably puts the nurse not only in the role of informing the chaplain when his or her services are required, but also in the first line for the meeting of spiritual needs (Cumming, 1993). Some patients may find it easier to talk about spiritual needs to a nurse rather than a chaplain, although others might value a visit from a chaplain or their own minister.

At the same time we realize that nurses are often faced with a predicament. While there are undoubtedly situations where the nurse is the most effective person to meet the spiritual needs of the terminally ill patient, they often do not have the time to spend listening in any depth when there are other tasks on the ward waiting to be done.

When one of the authors was at school playing rugby, there would be times when the ball would come out of a loose scrum and into his hands. His feeling then was one of panic, and his reaction to pass the ball on as quickly as possible. Nurses may share these feelings when spirituality is raised. Experience will teach the nurse when to deal with spiritual problems and when to call in a chaplain or other source of help. Hopefully, that same nurse will consider whether in fact he or she might be the best person to deal with the questions raised.

IDENTIFYING SPIRITUAL NEEDS

There appears to be an increasing recognition and awareness of spiritual needs on the part of the caring professions. As one of the people interviewed by the authors said, 'There is a greater emphasis now on religious and spiritual care, and what we don't know, we have to go and find out and ask.'

Some research has been conducted into spiritual needs and how they can be met and the findings have confirmed what is quoted above. Ross (1994b), for instance, found that 'of the 655 nurses who responded to a question on identifying spiritual need, 76.8% said they had identified a spiritual need at some point in their practice'. It isn't clear from this research, however, whether 'spiritual need' identified here was defined by requests to see the chaplain or other religious requests, rather than the nurse identifying spiritual need from the symptoms the patient was demonstrating.

As a result of this increased recognition and awareness, the UKCC have given guidelines for nursing practice. 'The United Kingdom Council for Nursing, Midwifery and Health Visiting (UKCC, 1984) states that it is the duty of the nurse to: "Take account of the customs, values, and spiritual beliefs of patient/clients"' (quoted in Ross, 1994b).

Nursing is not the only profession to take this on board. As quoted at the beginning of this chapter, Pass (1989), with reference to social workers' comments, 'It is essential to consider what spiritual care each patient may need, and to make it available to him, in response to his own unique need.' This attention to the spiritual needs of patients is particularly important when the patient is dying. Philpot (1989) states, 'The soul's preparation for death appears to require as much work, involve as much of a struggle, and demand as much realistic acknowledgement of the pain of dying as death's emotional adjustment demands. Spiritual preparation may therefore be described as the ultimate terminal problem-solving task.'

In order to help dying patients with their spiritual needs we must first identify what they are. We need to recognize how those needs may be expressed by the patient. Looking firstly at religious needs, there are various clues that might suggest that the patient might welcome a religious input. These include religious books or texts belonging to the patient, religious medals or statues, or religious practices such as saying grace before meals. All these things may indicate a religious stance in the patient. We must be careful, however, not to make assumptions about this. Questions as to what these things mean to patients will provide not only the information requested, but may well lead on to them speaking about their religious or spiritual needs. They may be helped by understanding that perhaps this is not a closed subject to the questioner. On the other hand, patients may express their religious needs in a negative way. Expressing anger against God, dwelling on their sense of failure or sinfulness, or a sense of fear may well be signs of religious or spiritual distress.

Spiritual needs not expressed as part of a religious faith are not always so easy to perceive. Statements about heaven or questions about an afterlife might seem like religious questions but they are often asked in non-religious ways, for example 'What is your idea of heaven?' or 'Do you think that there is anything after death?'

Other questions that might be asked are 'Why me?', 'Why suffering?', 'What are we here for?', 'What is the meaning of it all?' and 'How do you make sense of the senseless?' Spiritual needs may also be expressed in terms of statements rather than questions – statements like 'I can't see the point of going on' or 'It's all completely pointless'.

HOW CAN WE HELP TO MEET SPIRITUAL NEEDS?

The more that we have wrestled with spiritual issues ourselves, the more we can be of help to others with theirs. It is not necessarily the case that being able to give answers is helpful. Sometimes there are no answers. Answers that satisfy us may not be as helpful to someone else.

What helps a patient in spiritual distress is a willingness on our part to share their journey with them, to wrestle with them over issues of meaning and to help them to find their own answers.

In seeking to meet spiritual needs we are reminded that they are 'elusive and enigmatic' (Elsdon, 1995). This does not mean that they are beyond the reach of any sensitive carer.

Returning to the questions and statements referred to earlier, the patient's pain and questioning can be drawn out through a basic counselling empathic approach that does not seek to give answers but 'bears with' what is being said (Chapter 14). Some helpful techniques which may assist in the meeting of spiritual needs were discussed in Chapter 9. These include the use of touch to ease the sense of isolation that dying brings. Other things that have been found to be helpful include prayer (or the reading of appropriate prayers), reading – either the sacred book of the person who is dying or other religious books that they have found helpful in the past. Reminiscence can be encouraged. One nurse interviewed spoke of the use of aromatherapy, particularly the use of lavender oil, as a way of facilitating communal memories in a family. Talking about the people in photographs, or just remembering the good times, can be a source of solace and help. Finally, for many people music can be a very calming and helpful way of bringing peace. Patients, however, will guide us into the right way of helping if we are sensitive to what they are trying to communicate to us.

A wide range of religious, spiritual and cultural needs have been addressed in this chapter. It is hoped that the reader will have been helped to think more deeply about these issues. Also, that some ideas for improving practice will have been suggested. The following questions may help to address spiritual issues in practice.

Assessing spiritual needs

- What is the patient's current source of strength?
- In the past, perhaps at times of particular distress, has the patient found special help?
- How well is the patient making sense of his or her illness/suffering? How well are family members making sense of it?
- Does the patient have important concerns/things he or she is thinking about?

Coping with difficult situations

11

Death is the thing doctors are worst at. Thrust abruptly among the dying as students, they throw up defences, which are strengthened later as they become fearful of their own mortality. That is why they usually tell relatives, not patients – largely to spare themselves.

General practitioner quoted in Gathorne-Hardy, 1984

If the relative decides not to tell, it means that he or she has to lie to the patient from that time on and about a topic which is frequently on both their minds. The lie can create collusion right up to death . . .

Young and Cullen, 1996

This patient suspected that she had cancer but never said anything. Her husband thought she'd got cancer but didn't want to speak to her about it. Her five daughters and two sons thought she'd got cancer but didn't even talk to each other about it. And it was like this conspiracy of silence.

General nurse

Working with people experiencing loss inevitably leads to the professional helper having to deal with many difficult situations. Some of these will be referred to in later chapters, for instance having to cope with silence or denial after breaking bad news. In this chapter we will consider in more depth some of the difficult situations encountered by professional helpers focusing particularly on the problem of collusion and approaches to handling it.

First, as mentioned in Chapter 8, we return to the work of Glaser and Strauss (1965) on levels of awareness. Figure 11.1 represents their description of different types of awareness. A square indicates awareness, a dotted square incomplete or suspected awareness and the word 'and' means that there is discussion between the parties concerned.

In **closed awareness** the patient does not realize that he or she is dying but professional helpers and relatives do and they engage in a 'silent conspiracy' aimed at preventing the patient from finding out. **Suspected**

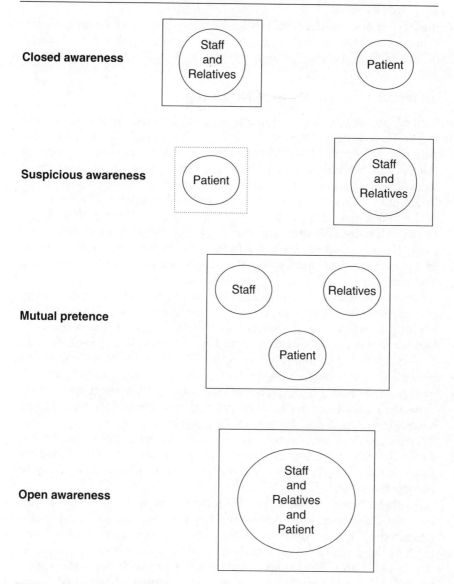

Figure 11.1   Levels of awareness.

awareness is when staff and relatives know that the patient is dying and the patient suspects this. In **mutual pretence** the patient, relatives and staff all share the same awareness that the patient is dying but they do not talk to each other about it. They pretend that the patient is not dying and that he or she will recover. **Open awareness** is when everyone involved knows the patient is dying and they openly communicate about this. Glaser and Strauss (1965) make the point that it is essential to understand the awareness context in which an interaction takes place because of its effect on the way patient, relatives and staff relate to each other.

SIMPLISTIC NOTIONS OF 'KNOWING'

Patients do not live in a vacuum, divorced from what is going on around them. They hear professional helpers talking about them and other patients. They may detect changes in the way professional helpers or relatives are behaving towards them. The former may, for example, begin to avoid them more and relatives may suddenly become more placid. Young and Cullen (1996) quote a cancer physician who noted that one of the major giveaways is that people stop arguing. Things that always caused a family row are completely ignored. Another clue that something has changed is when relatives who previously rarely engaged in physical contact start to do this, for example kissing on greeting and parting.

Some research studies indicate that people can 'know' even though this has not been openly expressed. Cartwright *et al.* (1973) interviewed cancer patients within a year before their deaths and found that 47% had some awareness that they would not recover. Centeno-Cortes and Nunez-Olarte (1994) found in a sample of 97 Spanish terminally ill cancer patients that 68% had not been informed of their diagnosis and that 60% of this group had a high degree of suspicion of their diagnosis.

As their condition deteriorates patients will probably have stronger suspicions or become more sure that something is seriously wrong. They may pick up non-verbal cues or make inferences from what professional helpers and relatives do not say; if, for instance, when they try to broach the subject of their illness their relatives jolly them along or change the subject.

All these factors make it possible for patients to 'know' even though they have not been told. An example of knowing before being told is described by Davis (1993). A registrar approached a couple to inform them of the probable imminent death of their son on a cardiac unit. He was hesitant and anxious and asked them about their fears and expectations. Their reply was that, although no member of staff had talked to them about it, they knew that their son had little time to live and he had already spoken of it with them.

WHY DOES COLLUSION OCCUR?

Young and Cullen (1996) suggest that doctors are more likely to tell relatives the bad news rather than the patient because they fear the response of the patient. They may be blamed for the bad news they bring or the patient may be more likely to get angry. Another fear is that if patients were told the truth they would be highly anxious or depressed and give up. A stronger way of formulating this fear is that the process of giving up would itself kill the patient. Linked to this is the notion that telling patients would take away any hope that they had.

Davey's (1988) study showed that some doctors, mainly surgeons, were reluctant to tell patients they had cancer. They assumed that patients would not want to know their diagnosis unless they asked directly. This applied particularly if the patient was elderly, working class and poorly educated.

As already discussed in Chapter 6, another reason why doctors may prefer to collude with relatives is that telling patients they are going to die is to be confronted directly with both failure and one's own fears about mortality. Mystakidou *et al.* (1996), in a survey of Greek doctors, found that their emotional reactions at the time of communicating a cancer diagnosis included sadness, anxiety and to a lesser extent guilt and fear.

When a relative wants to prevent a patient from knowing the truth, or *vice versa*, it could be construed as an act of love – an attempt to prevent the anguish that might be caused. On the other hand, it could be an indication that the withholder couldn't cope with the information being out in the open and having to talk about it. When a doctor tells a relative and not the patient, he or she may be conveying the message that the patient shouldn't be told or couldn't cope with being told, thus increasing the likelihood that the relative will collude.

Understanding the fears and false assumptions that can lead to collusion is a first step in beginning to address the problem. It is also helpful to consider the disadvantages.

THE COST OF COLLUSION

Imagine the following hypothetical situation. You have won a lot of money, only one friend knows and you are trying to keep it a secret from close family members. You would probably have to lie, for example to say that you couldn't afford certain things, and be very careful not to give any clues, such as buying anything that might be regarded as extravagant. If, say, you and your partner were experiencing any financial difficulties, you would probably have to appear (falsely) to be concerned. There might be many things that you could do and sort out if you were open. Even though this is a 'pleasant' secret, you would be likely to experience stress and strain from having to pretend that things hadn't changed.

Similarly, when patients or relatives keep secrets it can impose a high level of strain on them. Stedeford (1981) illustrates the psychological pain that collusion can cause. A patient in her late 30s with teenage daughters had a glioblastoma (a malignant tumour in the brain). Although this could only be partly removed, the neurosurgeon decided that she should be told that she had a cyst and that radiotherapy would cure it. Although the husband wanted to share the problem with his wife (which was their usual way of coping with difficulties), he felt he had to go along with the surgeon's decision.

Initially his wife thought she would get well because she made a partial recovery. However, after her condition deteriorated she became depressed and had suicidal feelings. By this stage her husband thought she wouldn't be able to cope with the truth and asked staff not to tell her, to which they agreed. As his daughters gradually became more aware of what was happening, they were forced to join in the collusion and 'all three of them found the tension almost unbearable'. The patient died frightened, confused and at times paranoid. Subsequently, her husband restated his wish that she had been told from the outset.

The only person who seemed to escape unscathed in this scenario was the surgeon. The patient was depressed and frightened, the daughters found it unbearable and the husband had strong regrets that his wife hadn't been told from the beginning. Furthermore, the patient had no opportunity to put her affairs in order or to finish unfinished business. Neither she nor members of the family were able to say goodbye to each other.

Collusion can also cause great stress for professional helpers. In the above example, we do not know the effect on nurses and other staff. However, in the following situation the effect on nursing staff is all too clear. A lady in her 60s was admitted to a medical ward following an extended cerebrovascular accident (stroke). She had previously suffered a mild stroke but recovered very quickly and returned to an independent normal life. During her rehabilitation this patient complained increasingly of headaches and drowsiness. Investigations revealed a secondary tumour in the brain. However, she was told that the diagnosis was only an extended cerebrovascular accident and, as she could move all her limbs, she believed that she would recover quickly just like the last time. The doctor spoke to the family and decided that the patient should not be told of her prognosis because she would probably lose hope and give up fighting. The family agreed as they were unsure of the best course of action and found it difficult to cope with the implications of the prognosis.

Nursing staff found it very difficult to evade the patient's questions when she asked about her condition and how long it would take for her to get better this time. It was noted that on some nights staff avoided her. As the patient's condition deteriorated nurses found it even more difficult to cope with her questions about why she was not improving. Overall nurses were uncomfortable and dissatisfied with this lady's emotional care, feeling that she was denied proper comfort and compassion. They thought she should have been told her diagnosis and prognosis from the beginning and found the whole situation extremely distressing.

This example also illustrates another cost of collusion: it can result in conflict between doctors and nurses and have a negative impact on team cohesion. This could in turn have ramifications for the care of other patients.

COLLUSION AND VULNERABLE PEOPLE

Some people who are more vulnerable or devalued than others are probably more likely to be on the receiving end of collusion. Children can quite often be 'left out' in loss situations. A training video entitled *That Morning I Went to School* (Pennells and Smith, 1991) ends with the following quote: 'At half eight I found out that my mum had died, by quarter to nine I was back at school.' One girl was not allowed to go to her mother's funeral. Her father said it might be too frightening for her. Instead she went to school. One child who was allowed to go to a parent's funeral said she was glad she went. However, she also wished that her younger sisters had been allowed to go and made the following insightful comment: 'If you don't go to the funeral, it's like you've never actually said goodbye in a way.'

In this general context of children's grief often not being acknowledged, it is perhaps not surprising that they can be subjected to some of the worst forms of collusion. A boy who didn't fully realize that his mother was dying wanted to visit her in hospital one day but his father wouldn't let him and she died the following day. Wells (1988) describes a situation in which a boy's father went into hospital for a minor operation and died under the anaesthetic. His mother couldn't bring herself to tell her intelligent 9-year-old son, who worshipped his father. Three days later, when friends finally told him about his father, his grief was overwhelmed by anger at not being told the truth. It wasn't until 5 years later that his anger and upset came out when talking to an understanding teacher.

Grollman (1990) describes how a college student reminisced about returning home from school when he was a first-grader to learn that his older sister 'had gone away and would not come back'. When he inquired what had happened and where she had gone, the response was, 'Don't ask so many questions.' For years he suffered recriminations, convinced in his own mind that he must have done something terrible to cause her disappearance. (This is an example of magical thinking, already referred to in Chapter 7.)

Another vulnerable group of people are those with learning disabilities. Oswin (1991) suggests that they may not be told the truth about a death because, for example, it is thought they would not understand or might cause difficulties for other members of the family or other residents in the institution. She mentions the care of a man who lived in a long-stay hospital and his elderly frail mother could no longer visit when his father died. Nobody told him about his father's death and for many months he worried (keeping it to himself) about what might have happened to his parents. Eventually he confided in the art therapy staff and, when they discovered that his father had died, they broke the news to him. He showed a normal bereavement reaction, including anger, denial and guilt.

Elderly people, especially those with dementia, may also be at risk of being kept in the dark. Maguire *et al.* (1996) asked 100 family members if their relative with Alzheimer's disease should be told the diagnosis and only 17 said yes. The main reason given for withholding the information was that it would depress or upset the patient. Paradoxically, 71 family members wanted to be told the diagnosis should they develop Alzheimer's disease. Maguire *et al.* (1996) suggest that family members may be protecting the patient from the harsh reality of the condition or be reluctant to deal with the patient's knowledge and possible grief.

An experienced nurse was caring for a male inpatient with dementia. This man had a fall and was taken to another hospital with suspected fractured neck of femur. At the same time his wife had a massive stroke and was admitted to the same hospital in an adjacent ward. His son (and his wife) kept this information from his father and later, when his mother died, also insisted that his father should not be told. The reasons given seemed to be mutually incompatible: that (1) he would not understand and (2) it would kill him. This man's wife had visited him twice a week for 4–5 years, so it was perhaps hardly surprising that he kept shouting for her. The consultant and the hospital manager joined in the collusion and forbade the nurse to tell. Even though this patient continues to ask for his wife, the collusion has been maintained for the 3 years since she died.

The common themes that emerge from this increased likelihood of collusion with different groups of vulnerable people include the following.

- They will not understand.
- They need to be protected.
- They will be too upset, which probably in reality means that the withholder will be upset.
- Their grief and their right to grieve is not acknowledged.
- They may not be told or involved because of their possible reactions.

A first step in reducing the occurrence of collusion with vulnerable groups is to accept them as individuals with the same needs and rights as everybody else. (Weeks (1990), for example, presents a bill of rights for children grieving because of a death, which includes, 'You have the right to ask any questions and receive thoughtful, honest answers.') Then we will be less likely to make assumptions about what they can under-stand and cope with and less inclined to protect ourselves from any ensuing distress they may show.

REDUCING THE PROBABILITY OF COLLUSION OCCURRING

The easier and perhaps customary route is to tell relatives first. In Mystakidou *et al.*'s (1996) survey 203 Greek doctors disclosed a diag-nosis of cancer all or some of the time. Of these 83% disclosed the diag-nosis and prognosis to the patients' relatives in the first instance. A first step in changing this process is to challenge it by asking oneself ques-tions such as the following.

- Why am I doing this?
- Am I making assumptions about the patient's ability to understand or cope?
- Just because the patient hasn't asked directly, does that necessarily mean he doesn't want to know?
- Does the patient suspect or 'know' anyway?
- Is it partly to make it easier on myself, so I don't have to face failure or my own fears?
- Am I anxious about how the patient may respond?
- What is the likely psychological cost to the patient, relatives and staff?
- Am I telling relatives because the patient is vulnerable or 'devalued'?

In early discussions with the patient the ground can be prepared so that subsequent collusion is less likely. For example, prior to any inves-tigations, the patient could be asked, 'Would you like us to discuss the results of these investigations with you on your own or would you prefer to have one of your relatives present?' It could be made clear that this is a routine question, so the patient doesn't jump to conclusions such as thinking that something serious must be suspected.

If patients don't ask questions about their condition it could be because they feel intimidated or less able to be assertive when ill, or that they perceive the doctor or nurse as not having the time. They might think they would not understand the medical jargon or that they will be told anyway if it is anything serious. So there could be various reasons why a patient doesn't ask questions on a particular occasion. Hinton (1980) found that, when staff were prepared for franker discussion, patients told them more and were more likely to disclose their awareness of dying. Developing a good rapport, being approachable, not using technical jargon and making it clear that one has time to talk could all help to facilitate more open communication. If, given these conditions, patients over a period of time never ask any questions and generally give the impression that they don't want to know, then it would be more justifiable to conclude that they are using denial as a coping strategy (see Denial – a troublesome strategy, below).

Another important ingredient in reducing the probability of collusion is team cohesion and communication. If each team member respects the others' roles and opinions then, for example, a doctor is less likely to make a unilateral decision that a patient should not be told. If medical and nursing staff are not sure about patients' ability to understand information concerning their condition, the views of other members of the team such as the speech and language therapist or clinical psychologist should be sought.

When patients develop a good relationship with a particular member of staff, they may be more likely to express their concerns and worries. This may lead to the realization that patients know more about their condition than the team thought they did. It may help to have a broad view concerning who can enlighten the multidisciplinary team. Schmele (1995) interviewed Ivan Hanson, a health-care professional for many years, who experienced a nearly 5-year struggle with cancer. He reflected on his contact with nursing assistants: 'I've had more pleasant conversations that were emotionally or psychologically healing with those people than I have had with the highest multi-degree medical professional.'

Other staff such as domestic or other support workers may also be important to some patients.

HANDLING COLLUSION WHEN IT OCCURS

When a relative requests medical or nursing staff not to tell, their reasons and feelings need to be assessed. Often there will be a cost to the relatives, including concern about things left unsaid, general stress and anxiety, as well as it affecting their relationship with the patient.

Faulkner and Maguire (1994) suggest that, having established the cost of collusion, a doctor could ask, for example, 'Have you ever thought, even fleetingly, that he (or she) may know?' Following a discussion about the possibility of the patient knowing, the doctor could negotiate permission to talk to the patient. The advantages of things being out in the open could be discussed and the relative could be reassured that only if the patient appears to know that he or she is dying would it be confirmed.

Once knowledge about the illness is openly acknowledged by all parties, the helping professional may need to bring patient and relative together. The patient may be feeling annoyed at not having been told and the relative may be feeling guilty. The helper may need to act as 'ice-breaker' in this situation.

One physician, when requested by relatives not to tell the patient, will say that if a patient wants to know, she is not prepared to tell a lie and so may have to tell the diagnosis. Importantly, though, she will also tell the relatives that she will say to the patient, 'We can help with "X, Y, Z"', so it is realized that all the patient's hope will not be taken away. If a relative wants to prevent the patient from knowing that another relative has died, this physician will first ask, 'Well are we going to be able to offer her the opportunity to go to the funeral?' The ensuing discussion will then cover the patient finding out at some point and his or her right to go to the funeral.

In the situation where both patient and relative know but are not talking about it, it can be helpful to have separate discussions with each. Sometimes patients will express the opinion that their relatives do not know of their awareness that the relatives know. Depending on the actual levels of awareness, appropriate negotiation could take place. One nurse commented that, if you offer to help, a patient may sometimes request, 'Well if you could tell her I know she knows . . .'

Sometimes a helping professional can act as a catalyst to help patient and relative break down collusion while all three are together. A general nurse described how this came about with a patient who hadn't previously spoken about her cancer and her husband. 'I stayed till gone 11 o'clock one night, she poured her heart out to me and told me why she thought she'd got cancer and that she didn't want to be left alone.' The nurse had to go home so the patient's husband came and sat with her. He stayed all night but she never once mentioned her fears. The next morning when the nurse came on duty the husband was still there and the following conversation took place:

Nurse: Have you told him why you are frightened?
Patient: No, I can't.
Nurse: Well, I think you should. (Then, giving some explanation to husband) This is why she's frightened, this is why I sat with her last night, this is what she fears.
Husband: Well, it's what I've thought for a long time.

Because the ice had been broken they were able to talk. The patient died 3 days later. At one level it could be argued that the nurse was being too directive. However, the husband must have suspected that his wife was very anxious if he was called to sit with her all night. Also, the patient clearly had a trusting relationship with the nurse and would presumably have felt able to request that the conversation didn't proceed to her husband 'being told'. Perhaps this nurse could have improved her approach by speaking to the patient on her own the next morning and asking whether she would like help in being more open with her husband.

A hospice social worker unwittingly acted as a catalyst when she made a home visit to complete income support forms with a dying man in his 70s. She had only just begun asking him questions on the forms, when he suddenly said, 'I'm going to die,' and then, 'I'm going to die quite soon.' The following conversation ensued:

> **Wife**: Oh don't talk so silly.
> **Patient**: Yes I am, much sooner than you think, and we've got a lot to talk about.
> **Wife**: (to social worker) This is all your fault – if you hadn't come here, he wouldn't be talking like this. Why did you have to come?
> **Patient**: Oh come here, just stop it and let's talk about this.

At this point the patient's wife burst into tears and so did he. She then sat on his knee. It would seem that the presence of the professional helper gave this man the confidence or courage to be open with his wife. Perhaps he felt safer that the social worker would be there to share the emotional turmoil. This is in fact what she did, even though she didn't say anything. Having acted as a catalyst and facilitated this important exchange, this worker left and offered to return to complete her original task. So sometimes helping to break down collusion may involve being in the right place at the right time and being prepared to listen.

Before concluding this chapter, we will briefly consider some difficulties caused by denial.

DENIAL – A TROUBLESOME STRATEGY

The reaction of denial after breaking bad news will be discussed in Chapter 13. In the short term, denial can be an adaptive coping strategy; it can protect someone from the full implications of what has happened. However, in the longer term denial can cause problems; for example, dying patients may refuse treatment which might help them. Also, if relatives deny that patients are dying it can lead to friction with staff. Denial can be a troublesome strategy in the sense that professionals may feel helpless with regard to the patient and relatives may accuse them of not trying. A hospice nurse described the reaction of some relatives: 'They hear about research on new treatments and think, because the patient can't have it, that we're not giving our best ... Also, if they visit and notice physical deterioration, it's "What have you done?" or "What have the doctors done?"'

There is an argument that, if a patient is using denial in the long term, it is his or her way of coping and s/he should be left to it. However, denial is not necessarily constant and there may be times when the patient's defences are lowered. Faulkner *et al.* (1994) suggest that it may be helpful to check for a window on denial by asking, for example, 'Are there any times, even for a second, when you are less sure that everything is all right?' If a patient seems to be moving in and out of denial, this could be pointed out: 'Yesterday you seemed to accept that your situation was quite serious but today you say you are going to get better.' The conversation that ensues will reveal whether denial is predominating. When their condition deteriorates many patients will not be able to maintain their denial. If a patient is able to move beyond denial, this opens the door to completing unfinished business and saying goodbye, as previously discussed.

A similar approach of looking for a window on denial or challenging inconsistencies could also be taken with relatives. Gently correcting misconceptions may also be helpful. In the example of relatives' reactions quoted above, this might include an explanation that research on new treatments can take a long time to translate into clinical practice. Also, they could be forewarned that they may notice physical changes in the patient.

Apart from feeling helpless when confronted with denial, professional helpers may also feel frustrated that the patient will not be able to die a 'good death'. It may be helpful to keep in mind that, for some people, denial may be the only way they can cope with dying.

In this chapter we have focused on the complex and difficult issue of collusion, including why it occurs and the associated costs. Ideas on reducing the probability of collusion and handling it when it occurs have also been explored. As Young and Cullen (1996) put it when referring to the practice of telling relatives instead of patients, 'Untold suffering must have been inflicted by this simple malpractice . . .' It is hoped that this chapter will assist the reader in helping patients and relatives to avoid such suffering.

How to break bad news

12

It is important to accept that you cannot soften the impact of bad news since it is still bad news however it is broken.

Maguire and Faulkner, 1988

The worst fear for doctors – particularly junior doctors – is that the patient will blame them personally for the bad news they bring.

Buckman, 1993

I'd have liked them to pay attention to me, and to find out what I knew and what I was ready to know.

The mother of a patient who had died

The breaking of bad news can never sound as if it were good news to those who have to hear it. What we can do is to minimize the effects of breaking bad news by the way that we give it. It is the aim of this chapter to explore ways in which we can improve our practice of breaking bad news.

Before considering the process of breaking bad news, we will present a few examples of actual situations where bad news has been broken badly.

HOW NOT TO BREAK BAD NEWS

A mother informed us of how in 1982 she answered a knock at the door to find two police officers standing there. One of them, having established that she was the mother, said, 'I am sorry to have to tell you that your son has been killed in a road traffic accident.' This lady has two other sons who are younger than the one who died. In October 1995 there was a phone call from the police. 'Your son has been involved in a head-on collision with a fire engine.' 'How are they?' asked the mother (she knew that her son was travelling in a car driven by a friend). 'They have been taken to hospital,' the police officer replied. 'Are they all right?' she asked. The response was, 'Oh, I don't know that. You'll have to ask at the hospital.'

One couple told the authors that their daughter had, while driving through a strange town, become involved in a road traffic accident. They had received a phone call from the hospital to come quickly. When they arrived at the busy accident and emergency department they were kept waiting for some time sitting in a crowded corridor. Suddenly a doctor appeared and told them that he was very sorry but the hospital had been unable to save their daughter. He then walked off again, leaving them alone in a strange place and without support.

Perhaps it is best that our final example is fictional. In the 1983 James Bond film *Never Say Never Again*, James Bond is dancing a solo tango with Domino in front of an admiring crowd. He suddenly and unexpectedly whispers to her, 'Your brother's dead, keep dancing.'

WHAT IS BREAKING BAD NEWS?

While the news that someone has died is very likely to be bad news, other situations also involve the breaking of bad news. Examples are being told that you have been unsuccessful in a job application, telling a child that his pet rabbit has escaped, redundancy, or the diagnosis of serious illness. Buckman (1993) defines breaking bad news in a medical setting as 'any information likely to alter drastically a patient's view of his or her future (whether at the time of diagnosis or when facing the failure of curative intervention)'.

With more serious news there is more potential for causing 'damage' to the recipient, so it is important that we break the news as well as possible. If it is important that we break bad news well, why is it that bad news is so often broken badly?

BREAKING BAD NEWS BADLY

There are many reasons why bad news is broken badly. We will seek to point out some of these.

LACK OF TRAINING

Thankfully, in recent years there has been a focus on breaking bad news and more training establishments are including it in their syllabus. This is, however, a fairly recent move. It is possible to break bad news sensitively without training, but training brings into focus important aspects and adds to what is learnt from experience.

LACK OF AWARENESS

Many professionals (medical or otherwise) have very busy schedules. They may find that many urgent demands are being made on their time.

This may lead to temporary tunnel vision. They may view breaking bad news as the next task, which needs to be completed as quickly as possible before moving on to the next one. This tunnel vision can lead to a lack of awareness of the needs of those who have to hear the bad news.

Lack of awareness can also include not having the micro-skills of interpreting body language, or distinguishing the nuances of inflexion, pauses or choice of words.

ANXIETY ABOUT PERFORMANCE

Breaking bad news is often a task that no one wants. Consequently the person breaking it tends to feel that, in Shakespeare's words, 'If it were done . . ., then 'twere well it were done quickly'. There is a temptation to get it over with as quickly as possible, in order to minimize the period of anxiety. This enables a quick escape from the discomfort associated with breaking bad news.

BUSYNESS

As has been written already under the heading of lack of awareness, the demands of a busy department, particularly Accident and Emergency, create pressures for doctors in particular to want to get on to the next thing quickly. This is especially so when what is done is not seen as being as important as the saving of lives or the treatment of the seriously ill.

PROBLEMS OF OUR OWN MORTALITY

Buckman (1993) outlines six fears doctors may have in breaking bad news. They include fear of not knowing all the answers, fears of the unknown and untaught, and a personal fear of illness and death. He writes, 'I would guess that doctors are just a little more inclined than the general public to believe that it can't happen to them. It's easier to keep this illusion alive by staying at a distance from someone to whom it clearly can happen and has happened.'

FEAR OF NEGATIVE RESPONSE

Even if bad news is broken well, we can never completely predict the effect this will have on those who receive it. Many of us find it difficult to deal with or even be in the presence of strong emotion. Faulkner et al. (1994) comment: 'The ancient Greeks always killed the bearers of bad tidings and the feeling that the bad news is linked to the carrier continues today.'

THE EFFECTS OF BREAKING BAD NEWS BADLY

People often remember bad news being broken to them badly many years after the event. Sometimes this can be long after other details about the death are forgotten, and the recollections frequently induce feelings of anger. Wright (1991) writes, 'It would appear that during this period of threat and distress we have a heightened or more acute perception of events.' Ashurst and Hall (1979) also write, "People remember vividly the way in which news is given to them, and they may go over it repeatedly through the rest of their lives. If bad news is broken clumsily or brusquely, their inevitable distress is greatly magnified, and they may be extremely angry.'

Breaking bad news badly can also hinder rather than facilitate the grieving process. The first task of bereavement counsellors often includes dealing with the feelings engendered in both patients and relatives because of the way that bad news has been broken.

In addition, the relatives may unconsciously reject information broken badly. As Maguire and Faulkner (1988) state, 'If you break the news too abruptly it will disorganize him psychologically and he will have difficulty adapting. Alternatively, it may provoke denial because the news is too painful to assimilate.'

THE EFFECTS OF BREAKING BAD NEWS WELL

We are aware that bad news can never be broken in a way that makes it welcome to the recipient. It can be given, however, in a way that helps the hearers to come to terms with it, or at least it can be broken in such a way that the damage is limited. We believe that there are certain key concepts in the breaking of bad news appropriately. Bad news is broken well when:

- those who receive it are treated with respect and empathy;
- we acknowledge the needs of relatives and meet them wherever possible;
- we give the information using appropriate language;
- we give the relatives time to assimilate the information and space to take it in.

IMPORTANT FACTORS IN BREAKING BAD NEWS

Before outlining a model for breaking bad news we will first give some of the reasoning that lies behind it.

Human beings tend to find it difficult to come to terms with death. People take it for granted that those they love will always be around and think that death is something that happens to other people. This is so even when they have already experienced death in their own family. There is a tendency to unconsciously block that which cannot be coped with. This is done either by selective attention or by a simple refusal to hear. If time and care are taken in the breaking of bad news this blocking can be avoided, at least to some extent.

If, in breaking bad news, information is given at a rate greater than that which can be absorbed, the relatives will not hear it. An analogy may help to illustrate this. Many modern houses have contact breakers in place of the old electrical fuses. When the current flowing through the circuit is higher than the contact breaker allows for, the circuit will be closed down. Similarly, when people become overloaded or overwhelmed with information they will 'switch off'.

RECEIVING BAD NEWS AND LOSS OF CONTROL

What may be considered by some as bad news may not be perceived that way by those who receive it. For instance the relatives of someone who has been suffering for a long time with a debilitating and painful illness may have as a first reaction a sense of relief that the person they love is at last free from suffering. (See the loss and value window in Chapter 5.)

The degree to which bad news is considered bad news by those who receive it is not something that can be measured solely by the information imparted. It also depends upon the feelings of those to whom the news is broken. This is why it is important to ascertain what the relatives already know. It is also helpful to find out what the relatives' attitude towards the bad news might be before we break it.

Receiving bad news can rob people of emotional control. When they hear news that is distressing about someone they love (or about themselves) they have a tendency to become emotionally upset. It is for this reason that privacy is so important and why, too, the careful positioning of a box of tissues and a bin can be so helpful. For some in our Western societies any display of emotion in public is considered inappropriate (the famous British stiff upper lip). In other cultures a verbal or demonstrative display of emotion is considered normal.

Receiving bad news can rob people of control in another way. When people hear something that is as potentially devastating as bad news they may feel that they are in danger of losing control. It can seem almost as if their whole sense of what is normal is being swept away on a tidal wave of disaster. This can be heightened if they feel that hospital staff are making all the decisions for them. This is why the model we give seeks to restore control to those who receive the news.

Finally under this section, it is helpful for us to know that relatives appreciate it when staff express their condolences to them. Clinical nurse specialists have reported to the authors that they had received several complaints that no one had said they were sorry that the death had occurred. In contrast, some relatives expressed how helpful it was when staff spoke of things that they remembered about the dead person.

THE SEVEN-STAGE MODEL OF BREAKING BAD NEWS

We move now to consider the seven-stage model of breaking bad news (Figure 12.1).

STAGE 1: STARTING FROM WHERE THEY ARE

There is an old joke about a lost motorist asking for directions from a country yokel. When asked how to get to such and such a place, the yokel thinks for some time before replying, 'If l were going there, l wouldn't start from here.' The joke revolves around the fact that the poor motorist has no choice but to start from where he is. In breaking bad news it is important to start from where the hearers are. This can be done by establishing what the relatives already know, either by asking them or, if we already have a relationship with them and therefore know what they know, rehearsing that knowledge with them. In doing this a shared platform of experience is established, a platform not only of knowledge shared but also of knowledge assimilated.

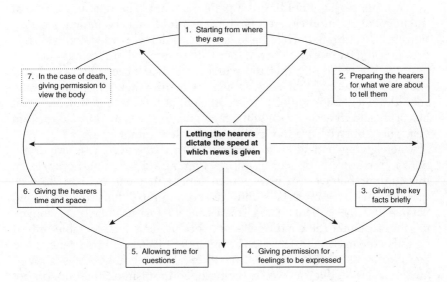

Figure 12.1   The seven-stage model of breaking bad news.

STAGE 2: PREPARING THE HEARERS FOR WHAT WE ARE ABOUT TO TELL THEM

A preacher, when asked what the secret of his preaching was, answered that he first told his hearers the subject of his sermon. He then gave them the content and finally, he repeated what he had already said. That illustration is a reminder not only of how little information is received when first heard, but also how important it is to prepare people for the information given. This can be done by using phrases that will 'flag up' the information that is about to be given. Television drama often uses the phrase 'You had better sit down'. Not only does this rob people of control by telling them what they ought to do, it also gives the bad news in too abrupt a fashion.

A better way would be to do as we have suggested and rehearse or find out what the relatives already know. Something like the following form of words could then be used: 'Since then his/her condition has deteriorated,' or, 'Things have not turned out quite as we had hoped/expected.'

STAGE 3: GIVING THE KEY FACTS BRIEFLY

Bad news has a tendency to overwhelm those who hear it. There may be a feeling that 'these things do not happen to me'. It is even more likely to overwhelm its hearers if too much information is given too quickly. It is important, therefore, to give the minimum information necessary and to give what else needs to be given, or is asked for, in bite-size pieces.

For example, a patient dies peacefully at 9.45 pm. A nurse is present at the time, perhaps holding the patient's hand. The relatives arrive at the hospital 10 minutes later, having been told that the patient's condition has deteriorated. They have come as quickly as they could. When breaking the bad news to them, there are several helpful things that can be said. We could say that the patient has died peacefully, that he or she was not alone, that a nurse was with him/her. This information should be held back initially. It is sufficient at this stage, following what has been said in accordance with stage one, to say something like, 'I am very sorry but you are too late. — died a few minutes ago.'

When giving bad news to patients or their relatives, it is important not to take away hope. For example, 'I am afraid we cannot operate on this tumour but we can give you treatment that will help to slow its growth.' Also, we must be careful not to minimize the situation either. Saying that the patient 'has a small cancer', for instance, may convey the message that the condition is not serious. This is acceptable only if what is conveyed is in fact what is intended. It is also important not to use euphemisms. Expressions like 'I'm afraid that he/she's slipped away' or 'He's gone', as well as being open to misinterpretation, do not help the relative to come to terms with the death.

STAGE 4: GIVING PERMISSION FOR FEELINGS TO BE EXPRESSED

Some relatives will express their feelings effusively and perhaps even violently at this point. Others will let go and then, catching themselves, will try to hold the feelings back. Others will be in shock and will register no emotion at all.

The purpose of the bad news interview is not to offer counselling. The need for counselling may become apparent later. At this stage the need is to acknowledge what the relatives are feeling and to give them back control by giving them permission to express that emotion. This may include offering a box of tissues to those whose eyes are filling, responding to a facial expression or body language by saying, 'You look as if . . .', or acknowledging their right to feel the way they do at this point by saying, 'I can understand your feeling . . .'

STAGE 5: ALLOWING TIME FOR QUESTIONS

Questions such as: 'How did he die?' 'Was there someone with him?' 'Did he suffer?' 'What do we do now?' are often asked. Sometimes people in shock may ask apparently callous or uncaring things, such as 'When can we take his clothes home?' or 'Did he have any money with him?' These questions arise from the relatives' inability to take in the meaning of what they have heard. Such questions need to be answered briefly and sensitively. The relatives need to be given permission to ask supplementary questions as and when they are ready.

Sometimes people are not able to take in all that is said at an initial interview. This is often the case when the bad news that is being broken is about a diagnosis. It is important, therefore, that they should be given an opportunity to return at a later date to ask the same questions again, or to ask others that did not occur to them at the first interview. A booklet containing the salient facts could also be usefully given at this point. Alternatively a tape recording can be made of the interview and given to them.

STAGE 6: GIVING THE HEARERS TIME AND SPACE

Bad news is always going to come as a shock, no matter how well it is given. Relatives need time in private before they are ready to face the world again. This is why it is important that, wherever possible, a room or office is used for the giving of bad news – somewhere where they can remain undisturbed before facing the world again. Many accident and emergency departments are now setting aside rooms for this purpose. A review report on early counselling of parents of children who were born with disabilities in Wales (Graff, 1989) reported that 'parents felt that after they had been told, they should be given a time to themselves in private – to talk, to cry, preferably with a nurse or someone they have met before, who can talk through their situation. Some parents complained of being given devastating news and then expected to leave the hospital immediately.'

STAGE 7: GIVING PERMISSION TO VIEW THE BODY

If we are breaking bad news that the person has died, permission should be given to see the body. (In the model this box has a broken line to emphasize that it refers only to cases where someone has died.) It is important that relatives are allowed to spend as much time as they need with the one who has died. Some people need to be assured that it is not morbid to do so. Others will need permission to touch or hold the person if they wish to do so. This may be particularly important when the death has been sudden or violent, as in the case of a road traffic accident. Wright (1991) encourages us to say to relatives: 'You can hold his hand if you want to,' 'Feel free to talk if you have things to say,' 'I am sure you want to say goodbye.'

Wright (1991) also tells us that 'it is important to see the deceased where they died . . . This somehow takes the bereaved closer to the event, and they have a strong need to be part of it.'

Before we leave the model, the reader will have noticed that it is circular. This is to remind us that breaking bad news is a task that sometimes has to be revisited. For instance, patients who have had the news broken to them that they have cancer, may need to be given more bad news as the illness progresses.

The reader will also have noticed that there are spokes radiating from the centre of the model. This is to remind us that breaking bad news is dependent not only on the information given but also on the relatives' ability to hear. Giving the relatives control over what is happening should also feature in how bad news is given. Wright (1991) says, 'People who have been affected by sudden death will talk about a loss of control over their lives and about powerlessness or helplessness.' How we give the news may either exacerbate or reduce this.

PRACTICALITIES

SETTING

We have already discussed some prerequisites for breaking bad news. We have considered the need both for time for the relatives to recover their composure, and for privacy. It is very difficult for them if they have to hear the news while standing in a busy corridor, or in a large ward where others may overhear or witness the news being broken.

Wherever possible bad news should be broken to relatives in a private room. It is preferable that the room has at least one window. This helps to relieve the sense of isolation that might otherwise be magnified by the feeling of being physically cut off from the outside world. It is also helpful if a note is put on the door indicating that privacy is requested.

If possible, relatives should be seated while the news is given. The person giving the news should also sit (on the same level, and not behind a desk!). Setting chairs at a 45° angle can be helpful. Wright (1991), writing of his research into sudden death, says, 'Most negative remarks were about the doctor not sitting on the same level when the news was delivered.' The person giving the news should not be distracted by notes but should make sure that he or she is in full possession of the facts before giving the news.

BREAKING BAD NEWS IN OTHER SITUATIONS

So far we have been discussing the breaking of bad news on your own territory, for instance in hospital. This is the most suitable setting, as factors such as privacy, space and the availability of other staff are within your own control. There may be times when breaking bad news in other situations is unavoidable.

BREAKING BAD NEWS BY TELEPHONE

One GP commented in this context that 'giving any bad news from a distance is not helpful'. Breaking bad news by telephone has several disadvantages. First, one has to be sure that the person who is on the other end of the line is the person anticipated. It is not unknown for bad news to be broken to the wrong person inadvertently!

Second, it is difficult to know the circumstances of people on the other end of the line. Are they on their own, or is someone with them? If someone is with them, is that person someone they would want with them at this time? Are people who can help within reach should they be needed?

Third, one secret of effective communication is the observation of body language. Unless, or until, telephones with VDUs are in common usage it is not possible to see how the person is responding to the news.

Some guidelines for breaking bad news by telephone

- Is this a suitable person to receive bad news by telephone? For instance, is there any reason to think that s/he might react badly to the news being broken? Is this an expected death?
- Are there any medical factors that make breaking bad news by telephone inadvisable?

- Is a support network known to be close at hand and available should the person need it?

When breaking the bad news the carer should:

- assess the current emotional state of the person (for example by asking how s/he is feeling);
- ascertain whether anyone else is present with the person – is this other person's presence likely to prove a help or a hindrance?;
- suggest that the person sits down while the news is broken;
- go through the procedure for breaking bad news, as outlined already;
- ask if the person is able to cope with what s/he has heard before ending the call (it may be appropriate to offer to telephone a relative for him/her);
- inform the person that s/he will be telephoned again later, and if at all possible do so within the next few hours in order to monitor their emotional state.

VISITING A RELATIVE'S HOME

Some of the problems that arise in telephoning are done away with when the person is visited for the purpose of breaking bad news to them. There are, however, other problems. The most obvious is that it can be difficult to give the news without interruption. People may enter the house without knocking, or the telephone may ring. Less obvious is that breaking bad news is never easy, even on the professional's own territory. As Manvey (1989) writes in the context of breaking bad news in a residential home, 'Most staff experience a feeling of panic at having to break the news of death to relatives.' It is even less easy when we have to do it on someone else's territory.

SUMMARY

In this chapter we have sought to draw the reader's attention to the ways in which bad news can be broken badly, and the effects this has on those who hear it. We have then sought to suggest ways in which bad news can be given more helpfully. Finally we have considered some of the settings in which bad news might be broken.

Lest all that we have written fills the reader with the sense of the impossibility of breaking bad news well, let us remind ourselves of the following points in conclusion. It is possible to break bad news in a facilitating way that respects the individual's needs at this particular time and helps rather than hinders them in coming to terms with the loss.

In breaking bad news the aim is therefore for the bearer to feel that, however distressing it was to give the information, it has been done in a way that respects the individual's dignity and has been done as well as it could be done.

Breaking bad news – the aftermath

13

I was asked by an ex-pupil (whom I know very well) to tell his girlfriend that his cancer had returned. He was 21, she 18. It was very difficult, she cried and I had to physically comfort her.

Teacher

Although I accept it as part of my job, I don't like breaking bad news. I always approach it with worry and fear and am anxious in case I say the wrong thing. I still don't know how relatives will react.

Surgery registrar

I find it very difficult to break bad news if I don't know the patient or the relatives because you can't gauge their reactions. You sort of sit back, impart the news and sort of wait for it.

General nurse

The authors' interview data and experience in training helping professionals suggest that there are common difficulties in dealing with people's reactions to bad news.

This chapter is divided into two parts. The first part will address problems that arise in those to whom the bad news is broken. In the second part problems that arise for the one who has to break that bad news will be considered.

PROBLEMS ARISING IN THOSE WHO RECEIVE BAD NEWS

DISBELIEF AND DENIAL

Disbelief and denial can appear to be the same thing. In fact, though they are closely related, they are different. Both responses are attempts to block information that cannot be contained at that moment.

In denial the person hearing the bad news simply refuses to accept what they hear. Buckman (1992) writes, 'The essence of denial is the patient's refusal to take on board the bad news, expressing the genuine belief that the news is not real or is a mistake.' A patient who asked a hospice social worker if he were going to die illustrates this point. When the social worker told him that it looked as if he were, the man responded, 'No, no, because it's convalescence, nobody's said, my wife's not said . . .' A consultant psychiatrist told us of another occasion when there was a very strong denial.

> We had a one-hour meeting; there was myself, a nurse, the patient's wife and son, and we broke the news that the patient had pre-senile dementia. The wife was not able to accept the diagnosis, she said the problem was secondary to a head injury and that her husband needed rehabilitation and why wasn't he getting it? She was offered a second opinion, which she refused. She made a complaint, which resulted in assessment by other staff. The whole process took about 16 months; only then did she begin to accept the diagnosis.

Our next illustration is one that demonstrates disbelief.

A senior nurse reported how she had visited a relative to break the bad news that her sister had died. She broke the news to her. The nurse then told us, 'I told her and I sat with her and then she just got up and did the washing up, and started cleaning the kitchen'. It was a few minutes before that lady could accept what had been said and she then began crying. In getting up and doing the washing up and cleaning the kitchen that lady was demonstrating disbelief, the inability initially to take in the information.

We can reduce the tendency for disbelief and denial if we follow the procedures for breaking bad news as described in the previous chapter. The more abruptly bad news is broken the greater the likelihood of disbelief and denial occurring.

It is important to differentiate the two terms because of the difference in the way that they are dealt with. Disbelief is a problem of taking in the information. Sometimes only time is required for the information to be received. With the lady cleaning the kitchen quoted earlier, the nurse reported that after waiting a few minutes the woman broke down and cried. Sometimes the relative may ask questions, perhaps the same question repeated until s/he is able to grasp the information. The important thing in this situation is simply to give time.

Denial needs to be handled differently. Denial is a natural and psychologically appropriate defence mechanism. As we saw in the quotation from the consultant psychiatrist, it tends to go on longer than disbelief. As the same psychiatrist also said in the context of presenile dementia, 'They need time to come to terms with the diagnosis; it is a gradual process and involves various members of the team'.

There are two fundamental errors to avoid when seeking to deal with denial. The first is collusion. It is tempting to go along with the denial as this avoids pain for both parties. Ultimately, though, it is not helpful to either. The other is attempting to force the pace in overcoming the denial. This may only generate anger for the one in denial.

The best way to deal with it is to refuse to collude with the person in denial while at the same time waiting for that phase to be over. (For more on collusion and denial, including looking for a window on denial, the reader is referred to Chapter 11.)

SILENT WITHDRAWAL

One of the most difficult situations helpers seem to have to cope with when breaking bad news is silence. Buckman (1992) writes, 'Perhaps the commonest symptom of shock is silence. The patient is simply unable to speak or respond to what you are saying.' Here are two situations that reflect the problem that this can cause for those who have to break bad news. 'For me somebody going quiet is the most difficult response to deal with. I think have they understood, why have they gone quiet, what are they thinking? Some ask to be left alone and I will go back later.' (Surgical registrar.) 'I find it very difficult when you impart the news and patients don't acknowledge it. They shut it out and may just talk about everyday things and I find it very hard to take the next step with them.' (General nurse.)

Wright (1991) explains the reason that nurses have difficulty dealing with silence. He writes, 'Nurses have great difficulty in seeing the value of just being there without putting it right. It is not like being able to put a bandage on and "making it better"'. What Wright (1991) says about nurses may have a bearing on other health-care professionals as well. Whatever the reasons for being uncomfortable, most people find it difficult when faced with silence in this situation. The great desire is to do something to 'make it better'. Perhaps the best that can be done is what might be described as 'masterly inactivity'. Sometimes it is sufficient to just be there. Talking, far from helping, can sometimes hinder the person who is struggling to take in the seemingly incomprehensible news that someone they love has died. Being with someone in their pain is often at least as effective as anything that might be said.

CLINGING

If silent withdrawal is found to be one of the most difficult situations for those breaking bad news, then clinging, as in holding on to the body, can be one of the most distressing.

One general trained nurse described how there was a very violent reaction to their father's death from two sisters. At one point she reported how she 'literally had to peel the eldest daughter off Dad's body. She threw herself on him on the bed.' She went on to talk about her regret at taking the daughter away from her dead father at that moment.

It is a very distressing thing to witness this prolonged clinging reaction but if time is given for relatives to come to terms with what has happened, eventually they will let go of their own accord and be helped by that experience.

INTENSE VERBAL RELEASE OF FEELING

This refers to several different verbal responses from screaming to wailing, from loud moaning to shouting. Such an experience can be very distressing for all concerned. One general nurse described a daughter 'screaming at the top of her voice' when she realized that her father was dead. A hospice nurse reported breaking the news to a family that a wife (and mother) had died. 'The little boy, who's got learning difficulties, had got this terrible cry: he threw his head back and wailed. It was awful and I felt totally inadequate. I wanted to cuddle him but he didn't want it'. Buckman (1992) points out that in some cultures people are more vocal than in others and screaming, shrieking or loud crying is more acceptable.

To be in the presence of someone making a loud noise is distressing to those who are there. It is also very distressing to other patients or relatives who may overhear. Consequently, it may be helpful to try to calm such a person down or, if this is not possible, to remove them to a part of the building where they cannot be overheard.

UNCONTROLLED WEEPING

This follows on from the last category. Copious tears can be very distressing to the people who are breaking bad news, not least because they feel in part that they are the cause. Tears are often a means of emotional release. Even if someone's crying seems to be out of control s/he will usually stop quite suddenly. If crying really does become protracted there might be a case for referring that person on for further help. As Buckman (1992) says, 'Some amount of crying may be part of the way a particular person copes with bad news, but prolonged collapse into tearfulness (say over several interviews over many days or weeks) is part of a more severe problem and is not a matter of "crying it out"'. We will discuss this in more detail in Chapter 15. To put things in perspective here, Wright (1993) tells us: 'Many people will want to cry and will need you to help them focus on the feelings that will help them begin the grief process.'

ANGER

'Doctors are far from perfect and on occasions patients and their relatives have reason to be annoyed with them, but such anger quite often
rises up when there is no apparent justification' (Hinton, 1972). Several
of the people we interviewed told us of angry reactions in those to whom
they had to break bad news. A staff nurse on an elderly care rehabilitation ward, referring to relatives, said, 'For some the death is so unexpected, they become very angry and you take the brunt of their anger'.
In the Warwickshire Police Unit video *Breaking Bad News* a man is
admitted for a routine hernia operation. During the operation he has a
heart attack and dies. A doctor has to break the news to his wife, who
has been waiting during the operation. When the news is broken the
woman responds: 'I – he can't have. He was here a little while ago. I
was just talking to him. He hasn't even finished wallpapering the sitting
room. If the bloody National Health had had him in 2 years ago when
he first started his hernia troubles this wouldn't have happened. Oh
God, what am I going to tell his mother!'

Incidentally, this last quotation also illustrates the way that people in
the first stage of grief appear to be thinking about seemingly inappropriate things, such as unfinished decorating.

Anger is a natural reaction to death. Colin Murray-Parkes has been
heard to say in a lecture that people have an expectation that disaster
always happens to other people. Even if a person suffers a loss in a
disaster where many around are suffering similar losses each will still
be saying 'Why me?'. This sense of being singled out can often result
in an angry feeling based on the perceived injustice of what has
happened. This anger may be directed against the person breaking the
bad news.

The important thing to do in responding to an angry response is not
to respond in like manner. To become angry oneself will only fuel the
relatives' or patient's anger. Realizing why people become angry when
bad news is broken to them enables the breaker of bad news to respond
in a way that diffuses the situation. To say to relatives that we understand why they are angry and that it is OK to be angry enables them
to ventilate their feelings harmlessly. Houel and Godefroy (1994), in their
book *How to Cope With Difficult People*, give three very useful pieces of
advice when handling difficult people. They suggest that we: (1) ask
ourselves whether their angry outburst could be justified even if we
would not have reacted that way; (2) take time to get our emotions under
control before responding; and (3) ask whether, in their words, they are
'just using the occasion to let off steam'. (These suggestions were given
in the context of dealing with difficult people in general. This last point
may not be applicable to a situation of breaking bad news.)

BLAMING

'In some ways it seems strange to deny natural death, by preferring to believe that the manner and time of death is the machination of some enemy or some power. However, men commonly wish to blame others rather than to acknowledge their own ignorance or personal limitations' (Hinton, 1972). Gunzburg (1993) speaks about clients using 'blaming language' and Wright (1991) reminds us that 'the professional ability or resources of individuals in the Health Service may be blamed'. This poses difficulties for those of us who have to break bad news. Comments like 'You should not have let him die' or 'You could have done more to save her' are sometimes heard. Earlier we quoted from a consultant psychiatrist to illustrate denial. Part of that woman's denial was to blame the medical staff for not doing enough. How are situations like this to be dealt with?

The first thing that needs to be established is whether there is any justification for the accusation. If more could have been done or if those who sought to help did not act professionally, then this would require investigation. If everything was handled appropriately, then a simple acceptance of what the person making the accusation is feeling, based on the understanding that this is a normal reaction to bad news, will often defuse the situation – a statement such as: 'I understand that you may feel that you want to blame us for what happened. Perhaps you would like to think about whether you wish to proceed further with this. If in the next day or two you still feel that way we can give you a copy of our complaints procedure.'

VIOLENT BEHAVIOUR

Sometimes the response to bad news is a violent outburst. One nurse described how the daughter of a person who had just died started head-butting the wall. More common perhaps are those who kick the door or start throwing chairs or other bits of furniture across the room. They may even threaten violence against the one who has broken the bad news. How can such behaviour be dealt with?

Buckman (1992) encourages us to stretch what we consider to be the boundaries of social responsibility when considering the response to breaking bad news. This includes pondering whether, in the peculiar situation in which hearers of bad news find themselves, the boundary of socially acceptable behaviour could be stretched. He also suggests that, when someone is behaving unacceptably, to respond calmly but firmly will usually result in the violent reaction losing its primary gain and it will resolve. If, however, the person is responded to in like manner, with rage or fear, this will only fuel the behaviour. As the book of Proverbs in the Bible says, 'A gentle answer quietens anger, but a harsh one stirs it up' (Good News Bible, 1976).

PROBLEMS ARISING FOR THOSE WHO HAVE TO BREAK THE BAD NEWS

Bad news is broken by human beings – by people who also have feelings that have to be coped with. Professional helpers are also expected to act in keeping with standards of professional behaviour. Having both to deal with feelings and conduct oneself in a professional manner can lead to various difficulties (see Chapter 3).

ANXIETY AND DISTRESS

In Chapter 12 we gave the example of the mother who opened the door to two police officers who told her that her son had been killed in a road traffic accident. This is an example of what we might term 'the hit and run approach' to breaking bad news.

A consultant physician we spoke to said, 'At the beginning when you first start having to break bad news, you're terribly anxious, you're very unsure of what you're saying and you're not very good at judging people's reactions.'

Part of the anxiety the consultant spoke about is not knowing how people were going to react and perhaps how an inexperienced person might handle that reaction. Another component might also be an anxiety about how the bearers of bad news might themselves react. It is the fear of inappropriate behaviour, or even that the bearers may not be able cope with it, that tempts them to break the news as quickly as possible and then withdraw.

A surgical registrar told us, 'I was involved in trying to resuscitate a child under 2 years of age, following a road traffic accident. The child died and I had to break the news to the family. They were upset and I was upset; I had to control my emotions at the time. I could have cried afterwards: I came close to it.'

One question we must all ask in this context is: to what degree should we allow ourselves to express what we feel? The cold, aloof, distancing techniques of the past are frowned upon now and we are encouraged to have a more empathic approach. As Buckman (1992) points out, the ideal we are encouraged to emulate is the unflappable hero like Clint Eastwood or John Wayne but, he says, 'when we break bad news, our patients expect us to have feelings of our own and we will appear to be cold-hearted and indifferent if we do not know how to deal with them'. But empathy means expressing our emotions. Where should the line be drawn if it is not drawn at no expression of emotion at all, as in the past? Buckman (1992) speaks of describing rather than demonstrating emotions, but he says this in the context of negative emotions like anger or frustration. Wright (1991) considers the display of emotion such as tears by the bearer of bad news to be an expression of sympathy rather than empathy, but is this so?

When is the expression of emotion appropriate and when is it not? There is no easy answer to that question. The guiding principle should be that the professional is there for patients and their relatives and not *vice versa*. The situation should not arise where the relatives have to comfort the carer. The professional's needs are best met by their colleagues offering appropriate help and support (Chapter 16). Where an expression of emotion facilitates the grief of others or demonstrates care it is, in the view of the authors, appropriate.

The words that follow come from a teacher and illustrate how her own expression of emotion helped the children in her class.

> I had to break bad news to the class when the little boy died and allow them to ask questions and talk about it. Many difficult questions were asked, including questions about burial, God and heaven. Because of my own beliefs and distress I found these hardest and tears came. They reacted to my tears (they trickled – I didn't allow myself to really break down until later when the children were gone) in different ways but several cried themselves for the first time (at school anyway).

In the next two sections we shall be looking at powerlessness and inadequacy in those who break bad news. We refer to powerlessness as those things over which we have no control, and inadequacy as those things we might or ought to be able to do something about.

POWERLESSNESS

Most people who work in the caring professions do so because they care. Their aim is to help relieve suffering and pain, whether physical or emotional, or to improve the quality of life for other people. Inevitably there will be times when this is not possible. Some conditions do not respond to treatment and the patient dies. Some conditions remain chronic, with little or no improvement. Inevitably this leads to a certain level of frustration. We can never do all that we would like to do. When faced with breaking bad news we can become aware of two things: first that we are the ones who are inflicting severe emotional pain on those to whom we break the news and secondly that we are powerless to do very much to alleviate that pain. Buckman (1992) describes this as 'therapeutic impotence'.

The situation may become worse if the person breaking the bad news has just been involved in trying to save the one who has died. Wright (1993) tells us, 'If a resuscitation attempt is unsuccessful and all resources were used effectively, it serves as a reminder of our scope and limitations.' If doctors and nurses, having been reminded of their limitations by failing to resuscitate, then have to break the bad news and witness the pain that this can sometimes cause, they may be left with a double dose of powerlessness. How can they deal with this?

It can help if we accept that being limited is part of what it means to be human. To acknowledge this enables us to take our feelings of failure and powerlessness and share them with others who can empathize with us. A sense of powerlessness can also be ameliorated if it is realized that in breaking bad news well we have helped to ease a situation that could have been made much worse.

INADEQUACY

Sometimes situations are faced that on reflection afterwards we know we could have dealt with much more effectively. One response is to feel inadequate and to try to avoid facing the same situation again. This leads to withdrawal, which we will be focusing on next. Another, more positive, response is to identify the needs for training and information and rectify the deficit when practicable. The potential usefulness of reflection as a support strategy will be discussed in Chapter 16.

DISTANCING OR WITHDRAWAL

Buckman (1992) writes, 'Some psychologists suggest that part of every health care professional's desire to be a doctor or nurse is, to some extent, based on a desire to deny his or her own mortality and vulnerability to illness.' (This may not necessarily be the case though – see Chapter 6.) The ability to fulfil this desire is seriously impeded when we are faced with patients who, for some reason, remind us of ourselves. This may be because they are of the same age or background. They remind us of ourselves or they have children of the same age or sex as our own. Faced with such reminders of our own mortality we may withdraw or distance ourselves from them. Buckman, again, comments, 'The commonest end-result of disliking a patient, or of feeling guilty, angry, frightened or ineffectual, is that you will withdraw from the patient. Withdrawal can be physical or emotional or both.'

Physical withdrawal is often seen in the avoidance of contact with someone who has a terminal illness. A surgical registrar speaking to one of the authors some years ago described how the surgical team would quickly hurry past the beds of those they knew to be terminally ill. They could not think of anything to say. Physical withdrawal is also seen in the desire to get the bad news out of the way as quickly as possible and to move on to something else.

Emotional withdrawal is more difficult to describe. It can be seen in the 'professional manner' in which some interviews are conducted; for instance, the brusque manner in which relatives or patients are sometimes addressed. Again, one of the authors remembers a time when his wife was seriously ill in hospital. He was visiting when the consultant physician arrived. He was asked to leave while the doctor informed his wife of the results of some tests he had ordered. The essence of emotional withdrawal is what Martin Buber called an 'I–it' rather than an 'I–thou' conversation. When this occurs we fail to meet with the patient as a person, but instead treat him or her as an object to be spoken to rather than entered into dialogue with. As Lake (1966) writes, 'As describing professional attitudes to patients or parishioners it [I-it] is a term which denotes the result of an impersonal attitude, disparaging the establishment of personal relationships between the doctor and patient, or the priest and parishioner'.

Buckman (1992) recommends that if we find ourselves withdrawing emotionally or physically we should ask why we are doing it and in our contact focus on those areas where we can offer something.

In this chapter we have looked at some problems that commonly arise out of the breaking of bad news. We have looked at some of the responses in those who hear that cause concerns for those who have to break the news. We have also looked at problems the breakers of bad news face in their own response. We have sought to offer some advice on how we may overcome these difficulties.

Adopting basic counselling skills

14

Please believe me, if you care you can't go wrong. Just admit that you care. That is really for what we search. We may ask for whys and where-fores but we don't really expect answers.

A student nurse who was dying, quoted by Ward et al., 1993

When people are in crisis, one of the first steps is to give them an oppor-tunity to fully express themselves. Sensitive listening, hearing, and under-standing are essential at this point.

Corey, 1991

In our experience the majority of patients and relatives seldom seek formal counselling from qualified counsellors but many want to talk over their circumstances with their professional carers.

Parkes et al., 1996

When considering the literature, we were struck with the degree of confusion associated with the word 'counselling'. The term is sometimes used to describe the giving of advice. However in counselling we should be cautious of any sentence we use that contains the words 'should', 'ought', or 'better' – as used in the phrase 'I think you had better . . .' All these terms represent the giving of advice, which is not normally subsumed under the term 'counselling'.

In other contexts people are said to be 'counselled' about their behav-iour – meaning in this situation that they are being disciplined for what they have said or done. Another view of counselling is described by Jacobs (1993): 'The term refers to a style of helping which emphasizes the client discovering his or her own solution to personal difficulties, without active direction or advice from the counsellor.' This is the perspective we will be using in this chapter.

Jacobs (1993) differentiates between the giving of advice and coun-selling. Being aware of the difference is important, particularly as giving advice can be costly. If you give advice that is good the client will rarely return to say thank you. If the advice is wrong you will almost certainly be criticized for it. In addition, in the giving of advice we rob the client of autonomy and control. These are among the very things that we seek to achieve in counselling. In terminal care, counselling may be likened to the process in which people who are floundering in the swimming bath are being helped to keep their head above water while they find their feet. It is important that people do it for themselves and that we only provide support and assistance.

Counselling is a way of listening and of asking questions within a 'safe space' that enables clients to explore their feelings and find their own answers. By a safe space we mean an environment created by the counsellor in relationship to the client in which the following conditions are met. First, that the client feels that the counsellor is on his/her side (**acceptance**). Second, that the client feels able to say anything s/he needs to without being judged or put down for saying it (**unconditional positive regard**). Third, that the counsellor is being 'real' with the client, and is not pretending to be or to feel differently from what they are trying to project (**congruence**). Fourth, that the counsellor conveys an understanding of what the client is trying to say (**empathy**). The reader who is familiar with counselling theory will recognize these as Roger's core conditions. (For more information the reader is directed to books on client-centred therapy.) In an unpublished MA thesis Whittaker (1995) asked non-nursing staff and volunteers who worked in a hospice about caring effectively: 'do you think that you need any special qualities or characteristics to work in this way?' The most frequent characteristics (and number of times mentioned) were as follows:

- the ability to listen (8);
- loving and caring (7);
- compassion (6);
- sensitivity (5);
- patience (5);
- understanding (5).

As can be seen from this list reported by Whittaker, the respondents came to similar conclusions to ours but based on their own experience.

Defined in this way counselling is an activity that is very broad. If we see counselling as a continuum, then one end of the spectrum takes place where a neighbour listens to another's problems over the garden fence. At the other end of the spectrum professional counsellors may practise psychoanalysis or one of the other psychotherapies. Figure 14.1 illustrates this.

People may employ counselling skills even though they are not specifically employed as counsellors. In the course of their work they find themselves at certain times in a counselling role. This may mean, for

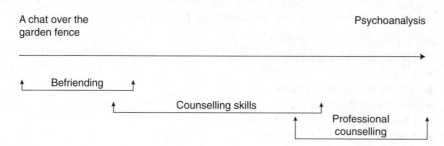

Figure 14.1   The counselling continuum.

some, counselling regularly but on only one occasion per person. So, for instance, nurses in an accident and emergency department may spend a considerable part of their time counselling people they will see only once. Others may find themselves counselling for a whole series of sessions, as for example, a nurse or social worker in a hospice. Longer-term episodes of counselling may also take place in community care settings, nursing homes or long-stay wards.

One staff nurse working in a psychiatric day hospital for elderly confused patients spoke of counselling as an on-going process. It some-times extended over several years as patients went through several stages of deterioration in their illness. She spoke of the many times on which she talked to one woman over the course of her husband's illness.

In talking about counselling we have used the word 'session'. In using this term we mean the length of time taken up with the use of coun-selling skills. This can be the magical '50-minute-hour' of professional counsellors. It can also be 5 minutes at the end of a nursing procedure, or words spoken to relatives as they are about to leave the ward.

We have already quoted Parkes et al. (1996), suggesting that most patients and their relatives seeking counselling help will look not to counselling professionals but to professional carers. This means that many working in terminal care will need to use counselling skills. Before looking in some detail at the purpose of counselling, we will outline some examples of unhelpful comments made to patients and their relatives.

UNHELPFUL COMMENTS

A hospice counsellor was asked to give examples of unhelpful comments that she had heard in the course of her work. She replied, 'It's all the things: "Time will heal"; "You've got to get down to building your life." I mean, there's just so many, it's unbelievable. Usually they're the things that have a semblance of truth in them.'

Whittaker (1995), in her unpublished MA thesis mentioned earlier, listed ten unhelpful sayings.

- Life is for the living.
- Time heals everything.
- You're doing really well.
- Keep a stiff upper lip.
- I know exactly how you feel.
- It must be the will of God.
- At least you're young and can remarry/have more children.
- It's time you were over it.
- You're lucky you had him/her for so long – you've had a good life together.
- You'll be fine – you'll soon get over it – time heals everything.

The reader may wish to refer to Chapter 5 for further examples of unhelpful sayings.

As mentioned above, there is an element of truth in many of these statements. What are people trying to do when they use these clichés? Often they are embarrassed and do not know what to say. They have heard these terms before and repeat them in the hope that they will be of some help. They may also see them as useful ways of putting an end to a conversation with which they are uncomfortable.

THE PURPOSE OF COUNSELLING

We have seen that counselling does not normally involve the giving of advice and it certainly does not include the offering of unhelpful platitudes. What then does counselling seek to achieve?

Worden (1991) gives four goals for grief counselling. He talks about increasing the reality of the loss and helping the person to deal with their emotions. (This means coming to terms with what they are immediately aware of feeling, but also recognizing those feelings that are not immediately available to consciousness.) The next goal should be to help the client to overcome various obstacles that are preventing readjustment to the loss, and finally to say an appropriate goodbye and to feel comfortable in reinvesting back into life.

What Worden gives us is the whole spectrum of bereavement counselling. (For more information on this see Chapter 7.) In terms of the goals of crisis counselling for the terminally ill and newly bereaved the focus is very much more in the shorter term. It is about helping clients to come to terms with what is happening/what has happened to them in the the present and the immediate past, and also to help facilitate the expression of emotion and to offer emotional support.

To return to the analogy of the swimming bath, to counsel is to help those who are floundering. It involves giving the necessary support to those who are struggling to come to terms with what is happening to them or has just happened. For some, much longer-term counselling may be needed, but that would normally be the responsibility of a professional counsellor or therapist. We will be considering this in more detail in Chapter 15.

BASIC SKILLS

Counselling is both an art and a craft. As with any art form the qualities that make for a good counsellor cannot be taught. Qualities like empathy, congruence and unconditional positive regard are very difficult to acquire if they are not innate. Most people, however, can be taught to be reasonably competent at any art form by learning the craft. In this section on basic skills we will endeavour to highlight aspects of the craft of counselling.

LISTENING

Most of us have been accused at some time of not listening when someone is speaking to us. When rebuked we often say, 'I am all ears' or 'You have my complete attention'. But the most attentive listening for most people falls short of what is meant by listening in a counselling situation. As Machin (1990) states, 'Listening is not simply a state of not speaking while another talks, but is a powerfully active engagement with the client's "agenda"'.

It might be helpful to think of listening not as a single activity but as a multiple exercise. Or, to put it another way, listening as we normally understand it can be compared to playing single notes on a recorder, while listening as a counselling skill may be likened to playing multiple notes on a piano. Listening in this sense involves listening to the words spoken and to the way that the words are spoken. This means listening to the intonation, to the relative loudness or softness of certain words and to the pauses and hesitations in what is said. It means listening to both the macro and the micro body language.

The macro body language refers to, for example, the clients' posture, the position in which they are holding their arms or what they are doing with their feet. Micro body language refers to the more subtle muscle movements the client might make. These may include a quick looking away, a fleeting smile or a frown. Parkes *et al.* (1996) call this kind of listening 'active listening'. They give a similar list to the one we have given above. They add, though, 'listening with our hearts to the human being we are trying to understand'. If this sounds very daunting to the reader, do not worry, as this kind of listening develops with practice. As Fish and Shelley (1983) say, 'Listening is an acquired skill.'

Guidelines to help facilitate effective listening

- Do not give answers. Clients are the experts on themselves and given long enough they will find their own answers if we create the right space for them. Parkes *et al.* (1996) write, 'Fortunately the very act of explaining ourselves to other people is itself therapeutic. While the bereaved are explaining themselves to us, they are also explaining themselves to themselves and this reassessment of life is one of the most important tasks of grieving.'
- Do not talk over. Only speak when you feel that it is necessary to help facilitate the client's own flow of words.
- Learn to distinguish silence that is embarrassing for clients from silence that is allowing them time to think. Ward and associates (1993) say, 'Listening is more than saying "yes" and "no" in the right places. People need space to come to terms with their feelings.' Of course that silence can go on for too long. If we sense that it is right to break the silence we can say something like: 'I wonder what you are thinking at the moment?'
- Listen for feelings. Words are only half the story.

Grollman (1987) quotes an unknown author as saying:

When I ask you to listen to me and you start giving me advice, you have not done what I asked.
When I ask you to listen to me and you begin to tell me why I shouldn't feel that way, you are trampling on my feelings.
When I ask you to listen to me and you feel you have to do something to solve my problems, you have failed me, strange as that may seem.
Listen! All I asked was that you listen, not talk or do – just hear me.

QUESTIONS

Asking a question is a simple thing, or is it? It is until you start thinking about it from the perspective of counselling. Counsellors talk about open and closed questions, intrusive questions, clarifying questions, controlling questions and so on.

Questions are best confined to those that encourage the client to speak: for example, 'Would you like to tell me about it?' or those that seek to bring clarification, such as 'I'm not quite sure what you mean by that: would you just tell me it again?'

It is generally unhelpful to ask closed questions, i.e. those that require only a one- or two-word answer. A counsellor might ask, for instance, 'Were you there when your husband died?' The counsellor should not be surprised when the answer to that question is simply 'yes' or 'no'. Whichever answer is given, it does not help the process very much and can easily lead into the next thing to avoid, interrogative questions, which are generally also unhelpful.

Questions that are interrogative tend to come one after another. If we did not know that the following was an example of a counselling session we might assume the client was being interviewed in a police station.

Counsellor: 'Were you there when he died?'
Client: 'Yes'.
Counsellor: 'Who else was there?'
Client: 'Just the nurse.'
Counsellor: 'Was that Nurse Jones you were talking about earlier?'
Client: 'Yes, that's right.'
Counsellor: 'And what did she say?'

We do not need to know what the nurse said. We can already see where this conversation is going and how we might feel if we were the client. The counsellor is being too intrusive.

How could this have been done differently? A question phrased as a tentative exploration might result in a simple no, but it will more probably result in the client opening up about his/her pain. An example of this kind of question is: 'I noticed that when you mentioned your husband's death you looked angry. I wonder if you want to talk about that?'

Another aspect of questioning is when the client asks us something. There are times when this is a straightforward matter. Sometimes, though, questions can be highly problematic. A hospice social worker spoke about the problem of a patient dying of cancer and someone in the same ward also having the same disease. She spoke of how one of these patients would say to her, 'That will happen to me, won't it?' This might appear to be a straightforward question, indicating that the patient wants a confirmation of what he or she suspects. But that patient might want to be told that his/her fears were groundless. How did the hospice social worker deal with this dilemma? She responded by putting the question back to the patient. What she said was, 'What do you think?'

If asking questions is a difficult area, then a much safer response is to reflect back to the client what s/he is saying. This is not simply repeating what the client has just said, parrot fashion, as the reader might have observed in some television caricatures of counselling. It means checking out what the counsellor perceives has been said by repeating it in his or her own words. Counsellors often use the phrase, 'You seem to be saying . . .', as in the following example from one of the authors' own experience.

Client: 'I am finding that I am not thinking about him all the time now.'

Counsellor: 'You seem to be saying that he is not always at the centre of your attention, that you are beginning to find that you are able to think about other things some of the time now?'

Client: 'Yes that's right. I'm not going over what happened in my mind all the time as I was.'

As we can see from this example, reflecting back not only enables the counsellor to judge that s/he has heard the client correctly. It may also give the client an opportunity to move on a bit further in his/her thinking.

NORMALIZING

Every loss is a unique event for the person who experiences it. People trying to cope with a major loss may not have experience of any similar event of that magnitude. This means that they have no 'maps' in their minds to reassure them that they are navigating or coping with their loss in a normal way. For instance many people express their fear of weeping. As one recently widowed woman said, 'I feel that if I allow myself to cry I'll never stop.' In the authors' experience of counselling weeping can be triggered by seemingly innocuous things like a touch, or the sight of a husband's pipe, or a wife's favourite scarf. When it starts, weeping can seem to be uncontrollable. When, unconsciously though, mourners have had enough they will often blow their noses and move on. When visiting one woman to arrange the funeral of her husband one of the authors experienced the widow breaking down and sobbing into her handkerchief for some time before wiping her eyes. She then said, 'I think I ought to make a cup of tea.' The weeping had stopped abruptly and she was back in control of her emotions.

We normalize when we reassure clients that they are not alone in what they are experiencing and that they will come through it. Whittaker (1995; quoted earlier) said, 'I think it's about everybody's journey being different. No one bereavement's like another. There are things that are common, but it's just take it as it comes, and have somebody check it out with you along the way, how you're feeling. It will get better. You will come through at some stage.'

When clients experience uncontrolled weeping it can be helpful to talk in terms of having 'an internal regulator that switches the crying off when they have had enough'. Another situation is where mourners experience auditory hallucinations of the dead person and they think that they are going mad. It is helpful to say something like, 'Other people have experienced that too, but it goes away after a time.'

Normalizing does not mean though that we dismiss what the client is experiencing as commonplace. Phrases like 'Oh, everyone goes through that' demean the mourner's experience and fail to acknowledge the uniqueness of that particular process for that person.

When clients' experience too closely follows our own there is a danger of our becoming **enmeshed** and attempting to normalize their experience with reference to ourselves. 'Enmeshed' is a counselling term meaning that we find it difficult to sort out what feelings aroused in us are empathic and which are the result of our own unresolved tensions. As one staff nurse working in long-term care said about her relationship with a patient's wife, 'I was able to relate to her loss. We were so similar ourselves and our husbands as well. It was difficult not to become emotionally involved, difficult to stay focused on **her**.'

GIVING PERMISSION FOR FEELINGS TO BE EXPRESSED

Different cultures have different rules about what emotions may or may not be expressed and at what time and place it is appropriate to express them. In Britain there is still largely the culture of the stiff upper lip. It is not generally permissible to express any strong emotion (except perhaps on a football pitch). Giving vent to our sorrow through tears is considered inappropriate in front of other people. This is particularly so for men. 'Big boys don't cry' is an expression that boys often hear from an early age. One feels tempted to add, 'But big men sometimes do.' In the same way, expressing our anger in any way other than verbally is also unacceptable. This is an area where women can often find difficulty. It is even less acceptable for women to express their anger physically than it is for men to do so.

Being aware of these problems, it can be helpful during an assessment session with a new client to say, 'Here is a box of tissues and a bin if you want to cry. If you do, I will just sit here and wait until you are ready to carry on. And here are some cushions. You can throw them, kick them or thump them if you feel the need to give vent to anger. Do what you like providing you don't do any damage.'

ARGUING

We have discussed before the way that anger can be a component in the picture we are presented with by the dying patient or the newly bereaved client. This anger can be very strong and sometimes misplaced. It can be very difficult to listen to someone giving an angry tirade against a colleague, particularly when we know it to be unjust or untrue, also not to respond if we are a person with strong religious beliefs and someone is railing against God. It is important that we do not argue in these situations. What is important is that clients are able to vent their feelings, irrespective of whether they see things correctly.

However, we do not have to agree with them! By saying things like, 'I can see that you feel very angry with — for what you feel to be their mistake/fault/lack of care, etc.' we are acknowledging the feeling and giving permission for it to be expressed, without making any statement about our own position on the subject.

Finally in this chapter we will give a short list of dos and don'ts in counselling.

- Encourage clients to talk. Remember, counselling is about listening, not giving advice.
- Don't talk over them. They need to talk, even if what they are saying is repetitious.
- Don't minimize the loss and avoid the use of clichés.
- Don't talk about trivia in the presence of the bereaved or dying. They will resent it.
- Do listen to what is being said and to what they might be trying to say.
- Learn to tolerate silence. Learn too to distinguish those silences that are helpful from those that are embarrassing.
- Question the temptation to reassure. Who are you trying to help when you reassure? Is it the clients or yourself?
- Don't argue with patients or clients. The important issue is what they are feeling, not the words that are the vehicle for that emotion.

In this chapter we have sought to outline some basic counselling skills that might be of help in counselling the dying and newly bereaved. We cannot during a single chapter give more than a few pointers as to how to develop counselling skills. The reader is recommended to read some of the excellent books on counselling that are now available or to consider getting some extra training.

Recognizing when further help is required 15

The socially isolated and those whose grief is complicated, need more intense help, and for longer.

Stedeford, 1984

We make assumptions that people will be all right, we have done our little bit, this is it, you have to go your way.
   General trained nurse, referring to the relatives of inpatients who have died

Seeking help is not an indication of illness. It's a sign of having the strength and determination to care well for ourselves.

Rubin, 1987

Implicit in the title of this chapter is the assumption that there will be times when it is appropriate to refer people who are dying or bereaved to other professionals.

DENIAL

We have written in previous chapters about denial in those who receive bad news, but professionals can also be prone to a denial of their limitations. There can be a temptation to regard oneself as omnicompetent. This can be associated with a feeling that we should be able to do everything ourselves and therefore not need to refer to outside agencies or other professionals.

A midwifery tutor spoke to the authors about a time when she tried to set up a self-help group for midwives. She attempted this because she and her colleagues had experienced a number of nurses coming to them individually for help with difficult situations. The group that was set up soon foundered for lack of support. When enquiries were made about why this was, it was realized that those who came to the group were labelled as 'wimps'. The philosophy of the staff in the department was that individuals should be able to cope with any situation that might arise.

A general trained nurse speaking to us about nurses' reluctance to refer people on to other professionals said, 'But I think we – maybe it's about relinquishing our power, feeling that, you know, we can do everything. You know, we can do the counselling and I don't – sometimes I think we're the wrong people.'

Parkes *et al.* (1996) underline the idea that there are times when it is appropriate to refer patients or clients in our care on to those who are professional counsellors. They write, 'It is clear that those caring for the terminally ill and bereaved need to have specialist skills to respond to the everyday situations they encounter. There are times when the added skills of a specialist counsellor are also needed.'

The question of competence in counselling is not the only issue. There is also the question of the appropriateness of counselling by those who have other priorities and calls on their time. Some nurses working in intensive care may be highly qualified counsellors in their own right. Being suitably qualified does not, however, make it appropriate for them to take from their work the number of hours that might be necessary to counsel someone effectively.

REASONS FOR REFERRING PEOPLE ON

When would it be appropriate to refer people on to other professionals? This is the question that we will be seeking to address in this chapter. We will first headline the reasons for referring people on, and then look at those reasons in more detail.

Indications of the need for further help in those who are terminally ill

- Anxiety
- Existential fear
- Prolonged silence
- Unfinished business
- Spiritual needs
- Disruptive or excessive behaviour.

Indications of the need for further help in the recently bereaved

- A history of not coping with previous bereavements
- A history of depressive illness, bipolar affective disorder or schizophrenia
- Suicidal ideation
- Inhibited grief
- Ambivalent relationship with the deceased.

Indications of the need for further help for the bereaved dependent on the nature of death

- Sudden death
- Suicide
- Death of a child – especially a grown-up child.

INDICATIONS IN THE TERMINALLY ILL

ANXIETY

A certain level of anxiety may be anticipated in those who are terminally ill. When anxiety levels become too great for the patient to cope with then something needs to be done. When it is found that either too much time is being taken up trying to deal with the anxiety or the help given is not sufficient, then further help needs to be considered.

Patients may show anxiety about the treatment they are being given, about whether they will be kept pain-free or about their breathing. Relatives may have similar concerns. All these things will normally be answered quite readily by the patient's nurse or doctor. It may be found that those anxieties are merely the presenting problem and that there are underlying concerns over relationships or the way that those who are left behind are going to cope. The latter issues may require more help than doctors and nurses are able to give at that time.

EXISTENTIAL FEAR

Cassidy (1992) writes, 'I believe that fear is universally experienced, at some stage, by those facing death. It may not be articulated and it may well not manifest itself in anxious behaviour, but it is there, at some level.' If that fear has to do with existential issues around the meaning of life and death or if the anxiety reaches overwhelming levels, then there may be a need to refer them on to someone else to try to help deal with these issues.

PROLONGED SILENCE

Silence is sometimes a means of withdrawing from society so that the patient may make sense of what is going on in their inner world. Most people find that a period of withdrawal from social contact for a short time can be beneficial. People in this situation may say things like 'I need a short time to myself'.

For some people silence can become prolonged as they become caught up in their misery. When someone is in a state where silence becomes unduly prolonged this may suggest that further help is required.

UNFINISHED BUSINESS

Where there is unfinished business people may not be able to die peacefully until it is resolved. They may need professional help to be able to do this. (See also Chapter 9.)

A staff nurse working in elderly care told us of an incident that occurred on her ward. She relayed how she spoke to the sister of a man who had died on her ward a few weeks previously. 'So his sister came up, and the reason she came up to see me was she wanted to know what I'd spoken to her brother about because he's haunting her. He's there in the morning when she gets up and he's there, he's with her all the time and there's something disturbing him.' This is an example of unfinished business for a relative which probably needed specialist counselling help.

SPIRITUAL NEEDS

This has already been touched upon when discussing existential fear, which is a spiritual need, but spiritual needs go beyond this, as was discussed in Chapter 10. Other spiritual needs related to guilt or the need for assurance may require specialist help.

DISRUPTIVE OR EXCESSIVE BEHAVIOUR

When people 'act out', when they express their pain or confusion in disruptive or aggressive behaviour, then they are not in touch with their feelings. They may need help to understand what is really troubling them.

Equally, when a bereaved person has problems with letting go of the one who has died, s/he may perform complicated rituals or turn the dead person's room into a shrine. This could indicate a need for further help. A consultant physician told us of a man of 80 who died of cancer of the rectum. He had a daughter of 45 and his wife had died the year before. The daughter was unwilling for him to come into the hospital in the first place. 'She didn't open up to anyone. She was strange from the minute she set foot inside the hospital ... Her whole purpose in life revolved around looking after father.' After her father died, she encountered the physician in the corridor and wanted to 'talk and talk'. A consultant physician does not normally have the time to listen to someone who wants to talk at length. That is the remit of other professionals.

INDICATIONS IN THE BEREAVED

A HISTORY OF NOT COPING WITH BEREAVEMENT

It may be found that in talking with those who are recently bereaved there have been other deaths that have not been mourned properly. It may be that circumstances dictated that they had to remain strong, or that family culture demanded a 'stiff upper lip'. If this is the case then the present bereavement may be doubly difficult to deal with. They may need help to give expression to their feelings or to understand what they are feeling.

A HISTORY OF DEPRESSIVE ILLNESS, BIPOLAR AFFECTIVE DISORDER OR SCHIZOPHRENIA

Any history of mental illness may indicate that the person may have difficulty coping with bereavement and it may be necessary to refer them to the appropriate services.

SUICIDAL IDEATION

Relatives may indicate that they do not feel they can carry on without the one who has died. They may talk about their thoughts on how they might go about taking their own life. Either of these situations is among the more obvious reasons for referring them on for further help.

INHIBITED GRIEF

Stedeford (1984) tells us: 'In inhibited grief the person seems to be very little affected by major bereavement, and the picture of typical grief never emerges.' Helpers who have longer-term contact with bereaved relatives will be in a position to observe inhibited grief. If this occurs, referral for additional help may be necessary to help the bereaved person move on.

AN AMBIVALENT RELATIONSHIP

Where an ambivalent relationship results in a conflict of emotions this can cause difficulties that may require further help to be resolved.

THE MANNER OF DEATH AND PROBLEMS THAT MAY ARISE

SUDDEN DEATH

Death tends to catch us unawares. It tends to come as a shock. When death is sudden (as with an unexpected heart attack) then the bereaved family might need to talk through their feelings with another professional. This is particularly so when the death results from a violent incident such as an accident or a murder.

SUICIDE

As noted in Chapter 1, feelings engendered by suicide are likely to be very strong and can include extreme anger. People bereaved by suicide may need further help to work through these emotions.

DEATH OF A CHILD

There is a sense in which the death of a child (sometimes the older the child the more difficult) feels to be an affront to the moral order. Children **do not** die before their parents. In an age where ideas of life after death are often confined to the investment of our lives into those of our children (as discussed in Chapter 6), then the death of a child is more than the dashing of our hopes for the future. Parkes (1996) quotes Gorer on the death of a grown-up child, as 'the most distressing and long lasting of griefs'. Ramsay and Unsworth (1995) tell us in the context of the need for support that 'studies and personal accounts have shown that this support is often lacking for parents whose children have died'.

So far in this chapter we have considered those situations where further help may be required. We have not discussed yet what kind of help may be needed or where that help may come from.

ASSESSING THE NATURE OF FURTHER HELP NEEDED

Additional help does not invariably mean professional counselling. There are many different needs that might require further help.

Before making any referral for further help an **assessment** needs to be made. Helpers considering this need for a referral may be able to make that decision on their own. Often such an assessment will take place in the multidisciplinary team. On other occasions a specialist such as a psychologist may be asked to make an assessment. This may be to ascertain both the need for further help and the most appropriate person or group for the patient to be referred to.

The need for further help may be as simple as ensuring that someone is with the bereaved person as s/he returns home. This is especially so for the first few hours for those to whom bad news has just been broken. One of the authors interviewed a general trained nurse. During the conversation the nurse realized that assumptions were being made that someone to whom bad news was broken in hospital would have support for the first few hours following their return home. She said, 'I suppose we just assume that we've done our little bit, they've done their little bit and now it's a parting of the ways, they're going to go home and they're going to sort things out.' Wright (1993) warns us, 'No one should leave the hospital alone as disorientation can be a problem immediately after such an experience.'

People who are dying are inevitably somewhat restricted in what they can do and their power to affect situations is limited. It may be difficult for dying patients to make their needs known. It may be even less easy for them to make contact with people they want to see, for example to write a letter to someone they care for. In such situations the need of dying patients is for **advocacy**.

Along with advocacy is sometimes a need for **practical help**. There may be a need for someone to check that the bills have been paid, or a need for someone to establish that the patient's house is secure. A patient may require someone to buy little necessities or to arrange the drawing up of a will. We must not forget that life goes on, even for someone who is dying.

As we have discussed before in the chapter on spiritual needs, there may be a need for **spiritual or religious help**. Patients or their relatives may want some ritual performed for them, to receive the sacraments or to be read to from a holy book. They may also, as we have discussed earlier in this chapter, have a need to discuss existential spiritual issues.

Finally in this section patients or their relatives may need **counselling** because they are having difficulty with a particular issue or because they are emotionally stuck. Worden (1991) writes: 'Today we observe that some people do not deal effectively with the tasks of grief and seek professional counselling for help with thoughts, feelings, and behaviours they cannot cope with. Others who have not sought out counselling directly will often accept an offer of help, especially when they are having difficulty resolving the loss on their own.'

SOURCES OF FURTHER HELP

When first considering sources of further help, we began with a fairly tight group including psychiatrists, psychologists, chaplains and counsellors. In considering this question, we have realized that many more people may be sources of further help. Below is a list of possibilities for referral. It is not meant to be exhaustive. Rather it is a list of suggestions as to where further help may come from that will hopefully trigger the reader's own ideas.

FUNERAL DIRECTORS

A general trained nurse when questioned about help with counselling said, 'I also ask them to contact the undertaker for bereavement counselling.' The authors' experience of undertakers is that they do not offer bereavement counselling. However in consultation with a local firm of undertakers it was discovered that some larger firms do offer information about the availability of counselling, but they are in a minority.

What all undertakers offer as part of their service is help in guiding bereaved families in the practical details they need to arrange following a death. They can be very useful in this respect. Some hospitals offer their own bereavement pack, which contains the names and contact numbers of local funeral directors.

A staff nurse on an elderly care ward told us, 'I always insist that, whether it's a post-mortem or it's a straightforward funeral-burial or cremation, they contact the undertakers that day. And I always point out that the undertakers are the ones who are more experienced in bereavement than we are and they can give all the practical advice that we can't.'

Other practical help may be obtainable from **solicitors** or **accountants**. If dying patients wish to make a will or to arrange their finances before they die, then these professionals may be useful sources of help.

ORGANIZATIONS

A number of organizations are able to offer professional help to those who are dying or recently bereaved. A list of some of these bodies will be found in the appendix at the end of this chapter. In addition to this there may be local bereavement support services that could offer help.

Another possibility for referral is to the primary care team within the health service. The team may be composed of palliative care nurses, psychologists, social workers or chaplains. Any of these people may be suitable professionals to refer the patient to. As Faulkner (1995), speaking in the context of social work, says, 'Usually social workers are less interested in the initial clinical assessment but will be called in later when other issues have been identified. It is sometimes easier to talk to someone without direct clinical experience as the interchange can be less threatening and more equal.'

Of course, effective referral requires that the relevant sources of help are known to those doing the referring and that an adequate communication system and procedure are in place. As Faulkner (1995) reminds us, 'communication with patients, families and friends will only be effective if the professionals communicate effectively with each other'.

In this chapter we have considered the principle of referring people on to other professionals and in doing so we have looked at possible denial of limitations in medical and nursing staff which may hinder this process. We then considered when it might be appropriate to refer on to other sources of help. We have looked at the nature of the help that might be needed and finally at possible sources of further help.

RESPONSIBILITY – A PERSONAL FOOTNOTE

In conclusion, one of the authors is reminded of a rule that he uses when considering his responsibility to the clients he counsels. He reminds himself that he is responsible to his clients but not responsible for them. In the context of this chapter this means that, as professionals, we are responsible for offering the best service we can to our patients or clients. This may mean finding appropriate sources of help to which they may be referred. We are not responsible for whether they take up that help or not. Ultimately, people are responsible for themselves (the exception is people with mental incapacity). Sometimes people are reluctant to accept further help, feeling that they should be able to cope or that seeing a counsellor, for instance, is a sign of weakness. Then what Rubin (1987) says may be helpful: 'There are many reasons why people seek professional help. Sometimes our friends aren't available to provide the kind of listening and support we need or we are troubled by the idea of burdening our friends.' Also: 'If a loved one of yours has been murdered or died a suicide death, if your direct negligence caused a loved one of yours to die, or if you've been raped or seen a violent death, it's best to talk to a professional person.' As mentioned above the responsibility of taking up our suggestions for further help lies with those who we are seeking to advise.

This was brought home to one of the authors several years ago when a young man was dying in a surgical ward in a local hospital. The author was asked to come in and try to help this man with his obvious spiritual distress and dis-ease and when he arrived, the man turned his back and would not talk to him. The sight of a clergyman at that time appeared to have too many connotations for him to cope with. The author left having learnt an important lesson. We can only help those who are willing and able to accept that help at that time.

APPENDIX 15A: SOME ORGANIZATIONS THAT COULD PROVIDE FURTHER HELP

Compassionate Friends
53 North Street
Bristol BS3 1EN
Tel. 0117 953 9639 (Help Line) Tel. 0117 966 5202 (Admin.)

Cruse Bereavement Care
Cruse House
126 Sheen Road
Richmond
Surrey TW9 1UR
Tel. 0181 331 7227 (Help Line) Tel. 0181 940 4818 (Admin.)

The Foundation for the Study of Infant Deaths
14 Halkin Street
London SW1X 7DP
Tel. 0171 235 0965
(Cot Death Help Line Tel. 0171 235 1721)

Jewish Bereavement Counselling Service
PO Box 6848
London N3 3BX
Tel. 0181 349 0839

Lesbian and Gay Bereavement Project
Vaughan Williams Centre
Colindale Hospital
London NW9 5HG
Tel. 0181 455 8894 (Help Line) Tel. 0181 200 0511 (Admin.)

Miscarriage Association
c/o Clayton Hospital
Northgate
Wakefield
West Yorkshire WF1 3JS
Tel. 0192 420 0799

National Association of Bereavement Services
20 Norton Folgate
London E1 6DB
Tel. 0171 247 1080 (Referrals) Tel. 0171 247 0617 (Admin.)

Stillbirth and Neonatal Death Society (SANDS)
28 Portland Place
London W1N 4DE
Tel. 0171 436 5881 (Help Line) Tel. 0171 436 7940 (Admin.)

Support after Murder and Manslaughter
Cranmer House
39 Brixton Road
London SW9 6DZ
Tel. 0171 735 3838

Support around Termination for Fetal Abnormality (SATFA)
73/75 Charlotte Street
London W1P 1LB
Tel. 0171 631 0285 (Help Line) Tel. 0171 631 0280 (Admin.)

Support for ourselves

16

The realization dawned that nobody at work was going to acknowledge my desperate need for time to reflect, to grieve for my father ... In re-donning the white coat, it seemed, I had covered up my claim to be a human being with the capacity to be hurt.

Junior doctor – Martin, 1993

Support from co-workers and peers is a crucial component of personal stress management ... only your co-workers and peers can provide the kind of empathy, feedback and encouragement essential to you as a helper.

Larson, 1993

Relations with family and friends are at risk if we expect such people to absorb the heaviest portion of our needs to debrief and discharge emotion.

Zerwekh, 1984

Much of this book is in a sense about supporting ourselves. Knowledge about common dying and bereavement processes can, for example, help to prevent taking angry responses personally. Understanding how professional expectations can be too high and insight into times of identification with patients or relatives can help to reduce stress. Feeling that one has some level of skill in such areas as breaking bad news or basic counselling will also lead to better coping. All these factors can play a part in more effective helping. However, perhaps the most important step in supporting ourselves is to acknowledge that working with people who are dying, bereaved or experiencing other loss is inherently stressful. This is illustrated by the following comments, the first from a social worker, the other two from teachers:

Working with dying patients and their relatives does take its toll. I come away sometimes feeling like a dish cloth, absolutely drained emotionally.

You have to be there for them in times of loss. I find that children take away my last ounce of emotional energy.

It was devastating to find 16- and 17-year-old lads coming for comfort following the deaths of their friends in a road accident. I went to the funeral with them, I felt I was supportive but needed a stiff brandy when I got home. I cannot remain aloof. I feel emotionally involved and it drains me.

From this, it follows that we should be respectful of our own needs, otherwise we may be sowing the seeds of eventual burnout. Apart from the latter being personally very detrimental, it would also mean that we wouldn't really be able to help anybody in loss situations. Often support may be viewed as secondary, something only to be concerned about if there is time. This attitude unfortunately devalues ourselves and our own needs and indirectly undervalues clients because it makes us less effective helpers.

This chapter will include consideration of various approaches to being supported, including formal and informal. We will also revisit some issues raised in earlier chapters, such as the importance of having a balance between working and non-working lives and generally supporting ourselves.

TYPES OF SUPPORT

As mentioned in Chapter 2, Pines and Aronson (1988) describe the following different types of support:

- having a good listener;
- technical appreciation, an expert who can give helpful feedback and appreciates your work;
- technical challenge, someone who can challenge your approach;
- emotional support, someone who will provide unconditional support;
- emotional challenge, someone who can ask whether you are perhaps not doing much work or maybe working too hard;
- shared social reality, someone who views things similarly to yourself, with the same kind of values and priorities;

Some of these kinds of support can be obtained informally, such as finding somebody who will just listen, while others which involve giving feedback and challenging are probably more appropriately provided in a formal way.

INFORMAL SUPPORT

Informal support is that which is obtained from peers on an *ad hoc* basis without prior arrangement to meet at a certain time or for a planned length of time. It is likely to occur in normal day-to-day interactions, particularly when chatting over a drink at break time.

A general nurse described how she sought out somebody who would listen and provide emotional support after a difficult interaction involving loss:

> I tend to find a colleague on the ward who I can talk to. I tell them how I feel I've handled it. There's one particular nurse, we take a coffee break and I'll talk to her. She's not qualified but she is just there for me. She sits and listens, she doesn't speak to me, she just listens and just lets me get angry and shout and get it out of my system.

Another nurse also referred to the value she put on support from untrained colleagues: 'They know when not to hassle you, when to make you a cup of tea and just when to be there.'

Perhaps these staff are good emotional supporters because they do not have the professional pressures and responsibilities of their trained colleagues. At times there may be difficulties with obtaining informal support, as illustrated in the following comment from a general nurse: 'The problem is getting time, getting somebody to stop and stand still. So sometimes you do go home bottling it up.'

Informal support may also be sought outside of work. In a group of teachers surveyed by the authors this source of support was used more frequently than support from colleagues at work. Off-loading was carried out with husband, other family members and friends. One teacher stated, 'I confide all my thoughts in my husband.' There are risks in relying too heavily on this kind of support, as the quote at the beginning of this chapter (Zerwekh, 1984) suggests. We may find that we need support in relation to our professional role at a time when our relative or friend is actually under more stress than we are. There are also issues of confidentiality to bear in mind and the ability of friends or relatives to understand one's professional role.

SUPPORT MAY BE NEEDED IN RELATION TO PAST LOSS EXPERIENCES

In training sessions with professional helpers, the authors have noted that many are able to recall a difficult loss, which can still be troublesome to talk about. Shanfield (1981) found in seminars with senior medical students and graduate nurses that old and unresolved loss and mourning experiences, both professional and personal, were reawakened.

The problem would seem to be that there has been no opportunity to properly process these experiences. The following is the recollection of a teacher concerning the death of one of her young pupils several years previously:

> One of my reception class died very suddenly from meningitis. I was devastated and his funeral remains in my memory as one of

the most painful experiences in my career. The tiny white coffin was so poignant. I can remember the real and physical pain of it all. Talking to the class was very hard indeed both before and after the funeral.

One of the authors interviewed this dedicated teacher and it was difficult for her to talk about this pupil's death. She was at times quite emotional and there seemed to be some unresolved feelings – for example, anger at the minister who conducted the funeral service. Although at the time of this traumatic event she had the informal support of a close colleague, she did not appear to have had the opportunity to emotionally process the experience (this will be discussed below under Debriefing).

A hospice social worker had the very stressful experience of a man having a fit and dying before the night was through, after she had broken the news to him that he was dying. He had insisted that he be told but was very shocked and had difficulty accepting the bad news. This worker's anguish was reflected in her statement, 'I searched my own soul ... could I have brought that on?' Although she had supervision, she liked to make use of informal support from colleagues at work. However, it was not until 12 months later that she off-loaded with a trusted colleague. This was partly because she was afraid that she had killed this patient and a colleague might also think this. Support would have been available had she asked for it. However, as she pointed out, it is not always easy to ask for the support you need: 'They're as busy as you are for a start and perhaps nasty things are happening in their lives, so you feel that you want to support them, not ask for support yourself.'

This example highlights the problems of relying too heavily on informal support at work. It also indicates again that people may carry unresolved issues about past losses that will need to be addressed at some point. This relates to the issue of accumulated loss or bereavement overload discussed in Chapter 4. Sometimes grief associated with past losses may be triggered off by current losses.

FORMAL SUPPORT

Support can be referred to as formal if it is planned and scheduled, and often it will occur on a regular basis. Such support can take place in groups or on a one-to-one basis.

DEBRIEFING

Debriefing is usually referred to in the context of traumatic incidents such as a major accident or disaster. It includes a meeting of both the people directly involved and those more on the periphery to review their impressions and reactions. Parkinson (1993) expresses the purpose as follows: 'The aim is to give an opportunity for people to talk and share their experiences and feelings, to reduce any after effects and also to minimize the possible development of symptoms of post-traumatic stress disorder.'

Post-traumatic stress disorder includes the occurrence of intrusive thoughts or images about the traumatic event, which can result in extreme anxiety or panic. Any reminders of the event are avoided. Parkes *et al.* (1996) suggest that post-traumatic stress disorder is more likely with sudden, unexpected and untimely deaths, especially if the survivor was present at the time.

It is easy to see how debriefing could help in some situations such as after a suicide or when people die a traumatic death, for example, with blood spurting about. However, it is our view that debriefing could also be usefully applied after losses that wouldn't necessarily be regarded as major or catastrophic. In the situation where a long-stay patient dies, many nurses and other staff may have known this person for many years. Some may have developed a close relationship with the patient. (An example of this scenario was given in Chapter 4.) A debriefing approach could be used to enable those staff to talk about the circumstances surrounding the patient's death and their thoughts and feelings. If no such arrangement exists for this kind of process to take place, as one nurse put it when referring to deaths on her ward, it is 'business as usual'. By this she meant that the usual pressures of providing nursing care continued and there was not time to properly acknowledge the patient's death. Lev (1989) refers to several articles that point to the value of a debriefing approach. Sheard (1984), for example, notes the critical importance of having a conference after a patient's death, so that staff can review their involvement with the patient and share their memories of him or her.

The process of debriefing, which usually commences within 2–3 days of the event, involves various stages that include discussing the following.

- **Reviewing the facts**. This includes exploring what actually happened and in what sequence. When and where did it happen? What did you do and say and what did others do and say?
- **Reviewing thoughts and impressions**. What were your first thoughts? What were your impressions and what senses predominate in your memory, e.g. sights, sounds, smells? What were your later thoughts, including any 'What if . . .?' or 'If only . . .' thoughts?
- **Reviewing feelings**. What were your emotional and physical reactions at the time and later? What was worst about what happened?

Sharing this kind of review can help people to appreciate that their own reactions are normal; in other words, that other people share their feelings, which might include sadness, helplessness and anxiety. Debriefing should be carried out by someone with some training in the process and this person should also have a source of support, i.e. someone to whom he or she can offload. A debriefing session could just be a one-off with participants pointed in the direction of further support should they need it. Another approach is for the debriefer to contact the people involved, say a month later, to discuss any continuing difficulties. The interested reader is referred, for example, to Hodgkinson and Stewart, 1991 and Parkinson, 1993.

SUPPORT GROUPS

Faulkner and Maguire (1994) describe the function of a formal support group as giving its individual members a chance to share the problems encountered in clinical practice and also to share feelings and reasons for difficulties in coping. The focus should be on generating solutions to problems. Unfortunately, setting up and running support groups can often prove problematical. Reasons include the following:

- The general work atmosphere (which is often influenced by the manager) is unsupportive.
- It is not considered sufficiently important to enable meetings to happen in normal work hours.
- The group is set up and led by a line manager, with whom group members may be reluctant to discuss certain issues.
- There are problems in finding someone to facilitate the group who is not part of the clinical group.
- Weak facilitation results in meetings just being moaning sessions.
- If only a small subgroup of a unit attend, this can create an 'in' and an 'out' group, with the former becoming territorial and the latter suspicious.

Nichols (1993) suggests that the vital foundation for an effective support group is a sense of 'psychological safety'. This can be achieved if attendance is voluntary and members feel safe in terms of status and confidentiality issues. Other ingredients for success include good preparation, so that members have the same understanding of what the group is for and what is supposed to happen. Practical issues include:

- group size – this should probably not exceed about eight people;
- ideally getting the same people to attend every time;
- frequency of meetings – probably at least once a month;
- having an 'outside' facilitator, i.e. someone with facilitation experience who is not directly involved in the work area of the group members.

Another important feature of such a group is that members can agree to contact each other in between meetings if anything distressing occurs. This might mean one member contacting one other member of the group after a disturbing event or a difficult day. As Nichols (1993) points out this then becomes 'a mutually supporting network which also meets as a group.'

In a small-scale study of 21 community nurses, Thomas (1995) found that two-thirds reported that attendance at a support group was of benefit in reducing the level of work-related stress they felt. Also, just under one-third reported improvements in self-awareness and their ability to put feelings into words. Llewelyn and Payne (1995), who use the term leader rather than facilitator, reviewed some studies of support groups for nurses and concluded that:

- they are likely to fail or be unhelpful if they:
  - are seen by those involved as having been imposed from above;
  - are focused on the personal emotional problems of the members;
  - are used by leaders or members for personal therapy;
- they are likely to succeed or be helpful if they:
  - are oriented around specific difficulties experienced in work, such as the distress caused by the death of a particular patient;
  - have an active, task-oriented leader.

In a questionnaire study of staff from various hospices Richman and Rosenfeld (1987) found, for example, that groups that offered technical challenge were more effective in reducing stress. When team members challenged one another this led to creative thinking, which could result in other strategies for intervention.

Sometimes support can be one of the functions of a group with a wider remit. For example, some nursing colleagues of one of the authors have formed a palliative care link group, which brings together representatives from different wards and hospitals. Its function is partly educational and involves professional updating but difficult practice issues are also discussed, thus introducing an element of mutual support.

ONE-TO-ONE SUPPORT

Getting support from another person on a one-to-one basis is probably what most often comes to mind when the word 'support' is mentioned. Individual performance review or an annual staff appraisal is usually carried out by a manager. The focus is on setting measurable and achievable goals, such as completing specific projects and attending training sessions. The danger is that adverse criticism will be higher on the agenda than giving positive feedback. The reader will recall an example of the former in Chapter 2.

There is a strong supportive element in one-to-one supervision, which may take place on a weekly basis or once or twice a month. Hawkins and Shohet (1989) describe the supportive or restorative function as helping supervisees to:

1. become aware of how the pain and distress of clients has affected them;
2. deal with any reactions.

They point out that failure to attend to these emotional reactions soon leads to less than effective workers. Other aspects of supervision are also supportive in a different way. For example, helping to develop skills, understanding and abilities (educative or formative function) can lead to increased confidence, which is in itself supportive.

The opportunity to reflect can be an important part of supervision. Boud *et al.* (1985) mention three stages of reflection: anticipating and thinking about an experience in advance; being aware of what you are doing while engaged in activities; and reflecting on and processing the experience. Fisher (1996) describes how hospice nursing staff used reflection to discuss how they felt about work experiences, how they handled them and what practice issues arose. This could then lead to considering changes in practice or policy. Shields (1994) reports on his experience of teaching nursing students to keep reflective work diaries on placement experiences, which were then discussed with a teacher. One of the student's comments illustrates the potential benefits: 'Reflection is like turning various ideas over in your head . . . looking at it from different angles . . . and realizing they meant a little bit more than you thought at the time.'

Duke and Copp (1994) make a strong case for the use of reflection in palliative care work. They describe the example of a palliative care nurse whose empathy and open expression of helplessness to a young, dying mother led to them crying together for 5 minutes. Reflecting on this incident, this nurse became more aware, for example, of the importance of being able to use her feelings in the process of care. For reflection to be helpful there should be a supporter who can be trusted to give both negative and positive feedback. Duke and Copp (1994) argue that reflection can lead to increased understanding: 'Reflection offers a powerful way to explore the interface between personal and professional experiences in practice. It provides a process for understanding how our personal lives mediate our responses to the demands made in our professional lives.' Such understanding can then lead to a reduction in stress at work.

PROCEDURES TO FACILITATE CLOSURE

Closure (referred to in Chapter 4) includes the process of acknowledging an ending, and this can facilitate grieving. In Chapter 9 some options for helping other patients to acknowledge a death were described; for example attending the funeral, holding a short service on the ward at the same time as the funeral, lighting a candle and having a remembrance book. These could also be helpful to staff. For those working in the community a follow-up visit to relatives at home or to speak to staff if a patient dies, for example, in a nursing home, can be helpful. Such a visit can help both parties to acknowledge the patient's death.

Davies et al. (1996) refer to closure as a process of 'following through'. In their study of nurses who cared for dying children they found that some made efforts to bring closure to their relationship with both the child and the family. They often stayed with the child until death occurred even if this involved working an extra shift, and 'after the child's death, some nurses followed through by making a special effort to talk with the parents or by attending the child's funeral'. This kind of approach to closure was seen as effective in facilitating the resolution of grief.

An awareness of the feelings of individual staff may be important. For example, in the situation where a professional helper has identified closely with a patient who has died or with members of the patient's family, it is probably more important for this staff member to attend the funeral or take part in an alternative service.

These things are probably more likely to happen if they are formalized, i.e. agreed with senior staff as normal procedures following a death.

Before leaving the topic of getting support from others it is worth noting its effects in the study by Davies et al. (1996) quoted above. They found, for example, that nurses who shared their distress were better at letting go, being there for the child and family, being honest and following through.

PROVIDING SUPPORT TO OURSELVES

The concept of support usually implies getting help from someone else, as discussed above. However, just as we can put ourselves under additional stress, we can also support ourselves. Some examples of self-support will now be discussed.

MAINTAINING A SENSE OF BALANCE

Riordan and Saltzer (1992), reviewing literature on burnout prevention, conclude that caregivers need to give special attention to their own efforts in forging a balanced personal lifestyle. The following questions may help the reader to assess personal levels of balance between work and non-work activities:

- To what degree is the boundary between work and home life blurred?
- Do I often work long hours?
- Do I have enough time for family and friends?
- Do I neglect pursuing interests and hobbies?
- Do I put off taking exercise because of lack of time?

Some professional helpers will do something physical if they have had a stressful day or week, such as going home and mowing the lawn, doing some weeding or digging, walking the dog or going swimming. The helpfulness of having interests outside of work was referred to in Chapter 2.

If one gets absorbed in the pressures that can build up at work, it is easy to lose a sense of balance or perspective. One nurse, whose partner had experienced life-threatening illness and survived, was going through a stressful period at work. She maintained a sense of perspective by telling herself, 'What I value most is the health of my family: at the end of the day the job is still a job.' Many professional helpers may have entered their chosen careers with high ideals and so view work as a very important aspect of life. However, it is probably more psychologically healthy to view work as **one** aspect of life and to consider that other parts of life are also important.

A sense of perspective can also be better maintained if we hold realistic expectations of our professional role. We will not be able to relate well to or help everybody. Some people may still have a 'difficult' death, however hard we try to enable a good death. (This relates to the issues discussed in Chapter 3 on being professional.) At the same time as maintaining this sense of realism, it is important to give ourselves a 'pat on the back' when things go well. This internal reinforcement (referred to in Chapter 2) can be quite significant as sometimes colleagues may find it difficult to give positive feedback, particularly if they feel under a high level of stress.

ENGAGING WITH AND DISENGAGING FROM WORK

Although an under-researched area, it is probable that rituals for connecting with and disconnecting from work may serve a preventative function and help to reduce stress. One nurse reported that when she went off duty she imagined leaving luggage at the ward door. This represented her work concerns, such as uncompleted tasks. Then, when going back on duty, she would 'pick up the luggage' and continue with her work. Warman and Fisher (1990) quote the example of a counsellor who would imagine putting a client's problems on a shelf, to be retrieved at a later date.

One of the authors, Callis (1996), carried out a survey of counsellors and found that methods of preparing to engage with clients included, for example, reading notes, preparing the room and relaxation. Disengagement methods included reflecting on a session and writing up notes. At the end of a working day, approaches to disconnecting from work included playing music on the way home and washing, then changing clothes. With respect to the latter, it may be that staff who wear a uniform at work can make an easier distinction between work and non-work clothes and hence find disengaging from work easier. However, those who are on call may find such psychological separation of work and home more difficult. One counsellor used visualization to separate herself from work; she imagined a sandstone wall between herself and client material. These simple strategies may help to prevent work concerns from encroaching too much on personal lives.

USING A RANGE OF COPING APPROACHES

Becoming overloaded with work can be the result of factors such as poor time management and an inability to say no or to delegate. Practice with setting priorities and being more assertive can be helpful. Generally, practising a method of relaxation can help to reduce stress levels (see e.g. Payne, 1995). As discussed in Chapter 2, people with certain kinds of attitude seem to cope better. They see things as a challenge, are committed to activities and relationships and have a sense of control. The more these kinds of attitude can be developed, the better one is likely to be able to cope with stress. Another form of coping is to recognize the limits of one's own competence and to seek further help for clients or develop one's skills. The issue of referring on was addressed in Chapter 15.

Although in some working environments it may be difficult to admit to stress, it can be helpful for a professional helper to say 'I can't cope'. One hospice worker reported that she could say to her colleagues, 'Look, this has been an absolutely horrendous week, I can't cope with much more of this. I'm going home.' This was not seen as a sign of weakness but as an indication that she was becoming overloaded with stress. Some organizations openly address this issue by having legitimate 'mental health days'. When somebody feels that stress is really building up they are entitled to take a day off to try to recuperate. It is generally found that this opportunity for respite is not abused.

Unfortunately, the authors are aware of some professional helpers who have not only felt undervalued but have also had their confidence undermined by more senior colleagues. This can be a very stressful situation that detracts from working effectively. Sometimes, in the interests of both the professional helper and his or her clients, the difficult decision to leave may have to be taken. As referred to in Chapter 2, more enlightened organizations will pay particular attention to involving staff in decision making and improving quality of care, as well as to formally recognizing their achievements.

One way to increase one's coping ability is to be proactive in trying to get the support one needs if it is not already available. Questions to ask in one's current job or of a prospective employer to ascertain to what extent staff are valued and a supportive environment is created, include the following:

- What kinds of formal support exist?
- Is the formal support available to staff at all levels?
- How is the formal support perceived by staff?
- Is there a systematic approach to staff development?
- How are staff involved in improving quality of care?
- How are staff achievements recognized?
- What communication is there between staff at different levels?
- Are staff clear as to how their role fits in with the aims of the organization?

In this chapter we have considered various aspects of support, including formal and informal, group, one-to-one and supporting oneself. The right kind of support is very important in enabling caregivers who work with loss to mature both personally and professionally. Harper (1977) described the maturing of the health professional in relation to working with terminally ill people. The final stage of this process is deep compassion, which is accompanied by caring based on humane and professional assessment of needs. We think it is appropriate to couch Rando's (1984) discussion of this final stage in more general terms, as it reflects the goal of effective helping, which has been the focus of this book: 'Caregivers are able to relate compassionately in full acceptance of the **person's loss**. Their behaviour and performance are enhanced by the dignity and self-respect they afford themselves, enabling them to give dignity and respect. The ability to serve another human being and to give of themselves manifests the caregiver's humanity to others.'

References

Abdel-Fattah, A. M. A., Benton, T. F., Copp, K. *et al.* (1992) *Helpful Essential Links to Palliative Care*, Centre for Medical Education, University of Dundee/ Cancer Relief Macmillan Fund, Dundee.

Adams, J. P., Hershatter, M. J. and Moritz, D. A. (1991) Accumulated loss phenomenon among hospice caregivers. *American Journal of Hospice and Palliative Care*, **May/June**, 29–37.

Ashurst, P. and Hall, Z. (1979) *Understanding Women in Distress*, Tavistock/ Routledge, London.

Autton, N. (1969) *Pastoral Care in Hospitals*, Free Church edition, SPCK, London.

Autton, N. (1996) The use of touch in palliative care. *European Journal of Palliative Care*, **3**, 121–124.

Barroso, P., Osuna, E. and Luna, A. (1992) Doctors' death experience and attitudes towards death, euthanasia and informing terminal patients. *Medicine and Law*, **11**, 527–533.

Bayly, J. (1969) *The Last Thing We Talk About: A Christian View of Death*, D. C. Cook, Elgin, IL.

Benner, P. (1989) *From Novice to Expert*, Addison Wesley, Reading, MA.

Beriman, S. L. (1991) *Facing Death: Images, Insights and Interventions*, Hemisphere, Washington, DC.

Bottorff, J. L., Gogag, M. and Engelberg-Lotzkar, M. (1995) Comforting: exploring the work of cancer nurses. *Journal of Advanced Nursing*, **22**, 1077–1084.

Boud, R., Keogh, R. and Walker, D. (1985) *Reflection: Turning Experience into Learning*, Kogan Page, London.

Bowlby, J. (1979) *The Making and Breaking of Affectional Bonds*, Tavistock, London.

Brewin, T. and Sparshott, M. (1996) *Relating to the Relatives: Breaking Bad News, Communication and Support*, Radcliffe Medical Press, Abingdon, Oxon.

Buckman, R. (1992) *How to Break Bad News – A Guide for Health Care Professionals*, Papermac, London.

Buckman, R. (1993) Breaking bad news, why is it so difficult?, in *Death, Dying and Bereavement*, (eds D. Dickenson and M. Johnson), The Open University/ Sage, London, pp. 172–179.

Buckman, B. (1996a) Cancer – what patients need to know. Lecture in Hanley, Stoke-on-Trent, UK, 23 May; see also Buckman, R. (1996) *What You Really Need to Know About Cancer: A Comprehensive Guide for Patients and Their Families*, Macmillan, London.

Buckman, R. (1996b) *I Don't Know What to Say: How to Help and Support Someone Who is Dying*, Pan Books, London.

Burnard, P. and Chapman, C. (1993) *Professional and Ethical Issues in Nursing: The Code of Professional Conduct*, 2nd edn, John Wiley, Chichester.

Callanan, M. and Kelley, P. (1992) *Final Gifts: Understanding and Helping the Dying*, Hodder & Stoughton, Sevenoaks, Kent.

Callis, S. (1996) An exploratory investigation into the experience of counsellors in engaging in and disengaging from counselling and the rituals they use to facilitate this. Unpublished MA thesis, University of Keele.

Cartwright, A., Hockey, L. and Anderson, J. (1973) *Life Before Death*, Routledge & Kegan Paul, London.

Carver, C. S., Scheier, M. F. and Weintraub, J. K. (1989) Assessing coping strategies: a theoretically based approach. *Journal of Personality and Social Psychology*, **56**, 262–283.

Cassidy, S. (1992) Terminal care, in *Cancer Patient Care: Psychosocial Treatment Methods*, (ed. M. Watson), British Psychological Society/Cambridge University Press, Cambridge.

Centeno-Cortes, C. and Nunez-Olarte, J. M. (1994) Questioning diagnosis disclosure in terminal cancer patients: a prospective study evaluating patients' responses. *Palliative Medicine*, **8**, 39–44.

Central Independent Television (1985) *Getting On . . . The Other Maggie*, (produced and directed by Keith Ackrill), Central Independent Television.

Clark, J. and Sister Jacinta (1995) The last hours of life, in *Caring for the Dying Patient and the Family*, (eds J. Robbins and J. Moscrop), 2nd edn, Chapman & Hall, London.

Collett, L. and Lester, D. (1969) The fear of death and the fear of dying. *Journal of Psychology*, **72**, 179–181.

Collins Concise English Dictionary (1992) Collins, Glasgow.

Cook, E. D. (1988) Existentialism, in *The New Dictionary of Theology*, (eds S. B. Ferguson and D. F. Wright), IVP, Leicester.

Cook, A. S. and Oltjenbruns, K. A. (1989) *Dying and Grieving: Lifespan and Family Perspectives*, Holt, Rinehart & Winston, New York.

Cook, J. and Wall, T. (1980) New work attitude measures of trust, organisational commitment and personal need non-fulfilment. *Journal of Occupational Therapy*, **53**, 39-52.

Cooper, C. L. and Cartwright, S. (1997) *Managing Workplace Stress*, Sage, London.

Corey, G. (1991) *Theory and Practice of Counselling and Psychotherapy*, 4th edn, Brooks/Cole, Pacific Grove, CA.

Cornette, K. (1997) For whenever I am weak, I am strong. *International Journal of Palliative Nursing*, **3**, 6–13.

Corr, C. A. (1993) Coping with dying: lessons that we should and should not learn from the work of Elizabeth Kübler-Ross. *Death Studies*, **17**, 69–83.

Cumming, A. (1993) Patients' access to hospital chaplains. *Nursing Standard*, **8**, 30–31.

Cushway, D., Tyler, P. A. and Nolan, P. (1996) Development of a stress scale for mental health professionals. *British Journal of Clinical Psychology*, **35**, 279–295.

Darley, J. and Batson, C. (1973) 'From Jerusalem to Jericho': a study of situational and dispositional variables in helping behaviour. *Journal of Personality and Social Psychology*, **27**, 100–108.

Dass, R. and Gorman, P. (1985) *How Can I Help?*, Alfred A. Knopf, New York.

Davey, B. (1988) Ethical framework of the consultation: doctors' assumptions about the patient's need to know. Paper given to the International Conference on Communication in Health Care, Churchill College, Cambridge, July; see also R. S. Downie and K. C. Calman (1987) *Healthy Respect: Ethics in Health Care*, Faber & Faber, London.

Davies, B., Cook, K., O'Loane, M. *et al.* (1996) Caring for dying children: nurses' experiences. *Pediatric Nursing*, **22**, 500–507.

Davis, H. (1993) *Counselling Parents of Children with Chronic Illness or Disability*, British Psychological Society, Leicester.

Deits, B. (1992) *Life After Loss: A Personal Guide Dealing with Death, Divorce, Job Change and Relocation*, Fisher books, Tucson, AZ.

Dickenson, D. and Johnson, M. (eds) (1993) *Death, Dying and Bereavement*, The Open University/Sage, London.

Du Boulay, S. (1984) *Cicely Saunders: The Founder of the Hospice Movement*, Hodder & Stoughton, London.

Duke, S. and Copp, G. (1994) The personal side of reflection, in *Reflective Practice in Nursing: The Growth of The Professional Practitioner*, (eds A. Palmer, S. Burns and C. Bulman), Blackwell Science, Oxford.

Eggerman, S. A. and Dustin, D. (1985) Death orientation and communication with the terminally ill. *Omega*, **16**, 255–265.

Elkins, D. N., Hedstrom, L. J., Hughes, L. L. *et al.* (1988) Towards a humanistic–phenomenological spirituality. *Journal of Humanistic Psychology*, **28**, 5–18.

Elsdon, R. (1995) Spiritual pain in dying people: the nurse's role. *Professional Nurse*, **10**, 641–643.

Etzioni, A. (1961) *The Semi-professionals and Their Organizations*, Free Press, New York.

Faulkner, E. (1995) The importance of communications with the patient, family and professional carers, in *Caring for the Dying Patient and the Family*, 2nd edn, (eds J. Robbins and J. Moscrop), Chapman & Hall, London.

Faulkner, A. and Maguire, P. (1994) *Talking to Cancer Patients and Their Relatives*, Oxford University Press, Oxford.

Faulkner, A., Maguire, P. and Regnard, C. (1994) Breaking bad news – a flow diagram. *Palliative Medicine*, **8**, 145–151.

Feifel, H. (1965) The function of attitudes toward death. *Death and Dying: Attitudes of Patient and Doctor*, **5**, 632–641.

Feifel, H., Hanson, S., Jones, R. and Edwards, L. (1967) Physicians consider death. Paper presented at the 75th Annual Convention of the American Psychological Association, Washington, DC.

Firth, S. (1993) Cross-cultural perspectives on bereavement, in *Death, Dying and Bereavement*, (eds D. Dickenson and M. Johnson), The Open University/Sage, London, pp. 254–261.

Fish, S. and Shelley, J. A. (1983) *Spiritual Care: The Nurse's Role*, 2nd edn, Inter Varsity Press, Leicester.

Fisher, M. (1996) Using reflective practice in clinical supervision. *Professional Nurse*, **11**, 443–444.

Florian, V. and Kravetz, S. (1983) Fear of personal death: attribution, structure and relation to religious belief. *Journal of Personality and Social Psychology*, **44**, 600–607.

French, J. R. P. and Caplan, R. D. (1973) Organisational stress and individual strain, in *The Failure of Success*, (ed. A. J. Marrow), Amacon, New York, pp. 30-66.

Friedman, M. and Rosenman, R. (1974) *Type A Behaviour and Your Heart*, Alfred A. Knopf, New York.

Fulton, R. (1979) Anticipatory grief, stress and the surrogate griever, in *Career, Stress and Death*, (eds J. Tache, H. Selye and S. Day), Plenum Press, New York.

Garland, J. (1994) What splendour, it all coheres: life review therapy with older people, in *Reminiscence Reviewed: Evaluations, Achievements, Perspectives*, (ed. J. Bornat), Open University Press, Buckingham, pp. 21–31.

Gathorne-Hardy, J. (1984) *Doctors: The Lives and Work of GPs*, Weidenfeld & Nicolson, London.

Gillis, E. (1993) A single parent confronting the loss of an only child, in *Death, Dying and Bereavement*, (eds D. Dickenson and M. Johnson), The Open University/Sage, London, pp. 274–277.

Glaser, B. G. and Strauss, A. L. (1965) *Awareness of Dying*, Aldine Press, Chicago, IL.

Glaser, B. G. and Strauss, A. L. (1968) *Time for Dying*, Aldine Press, Chicago, IL.

Goffman, E. (1959) *The Presentation of Self in Everyday Life*, Penguin, London.

Good News Bible (1976) Collins/Fontana, London.

Goodall, A., Drage, T. and Bell, G. (1994) *The Bereavement and Loss Training Manual*, Winslow Press, Bicester, Oxon. (NB In this manual the original source of the grief wheel is quoted as Grief Education Institute, Denver, CO, 1986).

Graff, G. (1989) *Parents Deserve Better – A Review Report of Early Counselling in Wales*, Standing Conference of Voluntary Organisations for People with a Mental Handicap in Wales (SCVO), Cardiff.

Griffin, G. M. (1990) Death: meaning, in *A Dictionary of Pastoral Care*, (ed. A. V. Campbell), SPCK, London.

Grollman, E. A. (1987) *Time Remembered: A Journal for Survivors*, Beacon Press, Boston, MA.

Grollman, E. A. (1990) *Talking About Death: A Dialogue Between Parent and Child*, Beacon Press, Boston, MA.

Grollman, E. A. (1995) *Living When a Loved One Has Died*, Beacon Press, Boston, MA.

Gunzburg, J. C. (1993) *Unresolved Grief*, Chapman & Hall, London.

Haight, B. (1988) The therapeutic role of a structured life review process in home-bound elderly subjects. *Journal of Gerontology*, **43**, 40-44.

Handy, C. B. (1985) *Understanding Organisations*, Penguin, Harmondsworth.

Hare, J. and Pratt, C. C. (1989) Nurses' fear of death and comfort level with dying patients. *Death Studies*, **13**, 349–360.

Harper, B. C. (1977) *Death: The Coping Mechanism of the Health Professional*, South Eastern University Press, Greenville, SC.

Hawkins, P. and Shohet, R. (1989) *Supervision in the Helping Professions: An Individual, Group and Organisational Approach*, Open University Press, Milton Keynes.

Hingley, P. and Cooper, C. L. (1986) *Stress and the Nurse Manager*, John Wiley, Chichester.

Hinton, J. (1972) *Dying*, Penguin, Harmondsworth.

Hinton, J. (1980) Whom do dying patients tell? *British Medical Journal*, **281**, 1328–1330.

Hodgkinson, P. E. and Stewart, M. (1991) *Coping with Catastrophe: A Handbook of Disaster Management*, Routledge, London.

Hollins, M. (1989) Things of the spirit, in *Last Things: Social Work with the Dying and Bereaved*, (ed. T. Philpot), Reed Business Publishing, Wallington.

Holmes, T. H. and Rahe, R. H. (1967) The social readjustment rating scale. *Journal of Psychosomatic Research*, **11**, 213-218.

Hopson, B. (1981) Transition: understanding and managing personal change, in *Psychology and Medicine*, (ed. D. Griffiths), BPS/Macmillan, London, ch. 15, pp. 323-348.

Houel, A. and Godefroy, C. (1994) *How to Cope with Difficult People*, Sheldon Press, London.

Hugman, R. (1991) *Power in Caring Professions*, Macmillan, London.

Hunkin, O. J. W. (1987) Religion, in *The Oxford Companion to the Mind*, (ed. R. L. Gregory), Oxford University Press, Oxford.

Jacobs, M. (1993) *Still Small Voice – An Introduction To Pastoral Counselling*, SPCK, London.

Jewett, C. L. (1994) *Helping Children Cope with Separation and Loss*, 2nd edn, British Agencies for Adoption and Fostering/Batsford, London.

Johnston, M., Tookman, A. and Honeybun, J. (1992) The impact of a death on fellow hospice patients. *British Journal of Medical Psychology*, **65**, 67–72.

Joseph, J. (1996) Warning, in *Poetry Please!*, J. M. Dent, London, p 54.

Joseph, S., Williams, R. and Yule, W. (1993) Changes in outlook following disaster: the preliminary development of a measure to assess positive and negative responses. *Journal of Traumatic Stress*, **6**, 271–279.

Kalish, R. A. (1985) *Death, Grief and Caring Relationships*, 2nd edn, Brooks/Cole, Monterey, CA.

Klass, D. (1995) Spiritual aspects of the resolution of grief, in *Dying: Facing the Facts*, (eds H. Wass and R. A. Neimeyer), Taylor & Francis, Washington, DC, ch. 10, pp. 243–268.

Kobasa, S. C. (1982) The hardy personality: toward a social psychology of stress and health, in *Social Psychology of Health and Illness*, (eds G. S. Sanders and J. Suls), Lawrence Erlbaum Associates, Hillsdale, NJ, pp. 3-32.

Kübler-Ross, E. (1969) *On Death and Dying*, Macmillan, New York.

Lagrande, L. E. (1988) *Changing Patterns of Human Existence: Assumptions, Beliefs and Coping with the Stress of Change*, Charles C. Thomas, Springfield, IL.

Lahiff, M. (1994) A basket of butterflies. *Paediatric Nursing*, **6**, 8–9.

Lake, F. (1966) *Clinical Theology*, Darton, Longman & Todd, London.

Larson, D. G. (1993) *The Helper's Journey: Working with People Facing Grief, Loss and Life Threatening Illness*, Research Press, Champaign, IL.

Lazarus, R. S. and Folman, S. (1984) *Stress, Appraisal and Coping*, Springer, New York.

Lee, E. (1995) *A Good Death: A Guide for Patients and Carers Facing Terminal Illness at Home*, Rosendale Press, London.

Lendrum, S. and Syme, G. (1992) *Gift of Tears: A Practical Approach to Loss and Bereavement Counselling*, Routledge, London.

Lerea, L. E, and LiMauro, B. F. (1982) Grief among healthcare workers: a comparative study. *Journal of Gerontology*, **37**, 604–608.

Lev, E. (1989) A nurse's perspective on disenfranchised grief, in *Disenfranchised Grief: Recognising Hidden Sorrow*, (ed. K. J. Doka), Lexington Books/D. C. Heath, Lexington, MA, ch. 25, pp. 287–299.

Littlewood, J. (1992) *Aspects of Grief: Bereavement in Adult Life*, Tavistock/Routledge, London.

Littlewood, J. (1993) The denial of death and rites of passage in contemporary societies, in *The Sociology of Death*, (ed. D. Clark), Blackwell, Oxford.

Llewelyn, S. and Payne, S. (1995) Caring: the costs to nurses and families, in *Health Psychology: Processes and Applications*, (eds A. Broome and S. Llewelyn), Chapman & Hall, London, ch. 7, pp. 109–122.

Lugton, J. (1987) *Communication with Dying People and Their Relatives*, Austin Cornish, London.

McGregor, T. S. (1990) Hospital chaplaincy, in *A Dictionary of Pastoral Care*, (ed. A. V. Campbell), SPCK, London.

Machin, L. (1990) *Looking at Loss: Bereavement Counselling Pack*, Longman, Harlow.

McMahon, R. and Pearson, A. (1991) *Nursing As Therapy*, Chapman & Hall, London.

Maguire, P. (1985) Barriers to psychological care of the dying. *British Medical Journal*, **291**, 1711–1713.

Maguire, P. and Faulkner, A. (1988) Communicating with cancer patients: 1 Handling bad news and difficult questions. *British Medical Journal*, **297**, 907–909.

Maguire, C. P., Kirby, M., Coen, R. *et al.* (1996) Family members' attitudes toward telling the patient with Alzheimer's disease their diagnosis. *British Medical Journal*, **313**, 529–530.

Manvey, C. (1989) Death in residence, in *Last Things: Social Work with the Dying and Bereaved*, (ed. T. Philpot), Reed Business Publishing, Wallington.

Marris, P. (1986) *Loss and Change*, Routledge, London.

Martin, J. (1993) Doctor's mask on pain, in *Death, Dying and Bereavement*, (eds D. Dickenson and M. Johnson), The Open University/Sage, London, ch. 17, pp. 83–84.

Maslach, C. and Jackson, S. E. (1981) The measurement of experienced burnout. *Journal of Occupational Behaviour*, **2**, 99-113.

Maslow, A. H. (1987) *Motivation and Personality*, 3rd edn, Harper & Row, New York.

Miller, D. (1991) Occupational morbidity and burnout: lessons and warnings for HIV/AIDS carers. *International Review of Psychiatry*, **3**, 439-449.

Mosby (1994) *Mosby's Medical, Nursing and Allied Health Dictionary*, 4th edn, (eds K. N. Anderson (revision ed.), L. E. Anderson (consulting ed. and writer) and W. E. Glanze (consulting and pronunciation ed.)), C. V. Mosby, London.

Moscrop, J. (1995) Looking at death and dying, in *Caring for the Dying Patient and the Family*, 3rd edn, (eds J. Robbins and J. Moscrop), Chapman & Hall, London.

Mystakidou, K., Liossi, C., Vlachos, L. and Papadimitriou, J. (1996) Disclosure of diagnostic information to cancer patients in Greece. *Palliative Medicine*, **10**, 195–200.

Neimeyer, R. A. and Van Brunt, D. (1995) Death anxiety, in *Dying: Facing the Facts*, (eds H. Wass and R. A. Neimeyer), Taylor & Francis, Washington, DC, ch. 3, pp. 49–88.

Neuberger, J. (1987) *Caring for Dying People of Different Faiths*, Austin Cornish, London.

Neugarten, B. (1972) Personality and the ageing process. *Gerontologist*, **12**, 9–15.

Nichols, K. A. (1993) *Psychological Care in Physical Illness*, 2nd edn, Chapman & Hall, London.

Nimock, M. J. A., Webb, L. and Connell, J. R. (1987) Communication and the terminally ill: a theoretical model. *Death Studies*, **11**, 323–344.

Older, J. (1982) *Touching Is Healing*, Stein & Day, New York.

Oltjenbruns, K. (1987) Impact of loss on surviving relationships: the 'incremental grief phenomenon'. Unpublished manuscript, Colorado State University, Fort Collins, CO; see also Cook and Oltjenbruns, 1989, ch. 3, pp. 90–129.

Open University (1992) *Death and Dying Workbook 1: Life and Death*, Open University Press, Milton Keynes, pp 11–12 and audiotape on facing loss.

Oswin, M. (1991) *Am I Allowed to Cry: A Study of Bereavement Amongst People Who Have Learning Difficulties*, Souvenir Press, London.

Parkes, C. M. (1996) *Bereavement: Studies of Grief in Adult Life*, 3rd edn, Routledge, London.

Parkes, C. M., Relf, M. and Couldrick, A. (1996) *Counselling in Terminal Care And Bereavement*, British Psychological Society Books, Leicester.

Parkes, C. M., Stevenson-Hinde, J. and Marris, P. (eds) (1991) *Attachment Across the Life Cycle*, Routledge, London.

Parkinson, F. (1993) *Post-Trauma Stress*, Sheldon Press, London.

Pass, S. (1989) An overview, in *Last Things: Social Work with the Dying and Bereaved*, (ed. T. Philpot), Reed Business Publishing, Wallington.

Payne, R. A. (1995) *Relaxation Techniques: A Practical Handbook for the Health Care Professional*, Churchill Livingstone, Edinburgh.

Payne, S. A., Langley-Evans and Hillier, R. (1996) Perceptions of a 'good' death: a comparative study of the views of hospice staff and patients. *Palliative Medicine*, **10**, 307–312.

Peberdy, A. (1993) Spiritual care of dying people, in *Death, Dying and Bereavement*, (eds D. Dickenson and M. Johnson), The Open University/Sage, London, pp. 219–223.

Pennells, M. and Smith, S. (devisors) (1991) *That Morning I Went to School . . . Bereavement and Children* (video), (producers S. Bownass and F. Palmer), Video Communication Services, Northampton.

Penson, J. (1990) *Bereavement: A Guide for Nurses*, Chapman & Hall, London.

Philpot, T. (ed.) (1989) *Last Things: Social Work with the Dying and Bereaved*, Reed Business Publishing, Wallington.

Pines, A. (1982) Helpers' motivation and the burnout syndrome, in *Basic Processes in Helping Relationships*, (ed. T. A. Wills), Academic Press, London.

Pines, A. M. and Aronson, E. (1988) *Career Burnout: Causes and Cures*, Free Press, New York.

Potter, P. A. and Perry, A. G. (1993) *Fundamentals of Nursing: Concepts, Process and Practice*, 3rd edn, Mosby, St Louis, MO.

Quoist, M. (1965) *The Christian Response*, Gill & Macmillan, Dublin.

Ramsay, J. and Unsworth, S. (1995) Care for the dying patient and the family, in *Caring for the Dying Patient and the Family*, 3rd edn, (eds J. Robbins and J. Moscrop), Chapman & Hall, London.

Rando, T. A. (1984) *Grief, Dying and Death. Clinical Interventions for Caregivers*, Research Press, Champaign, IL.

Richman, J. and Rosenfeld, L. (1987) Stress reduction for hospice workers: a support group model. *Hospice Journal*, **3**, 205–221.

Riordan, R. J. and Saltzer, S. K. (1992) Burnout prevention among health care providers working with the terminally ill: a literature review. *Omega*, **25**, 17–24.

Roberty, M. (1995) *The Complete Guide to the Music of Eric Clapton*, Omnibus Press, London.

Ross, L. (1994a) Spiritual care: the nurse's role. *Nursing Standard*, **8**, 33–37.

Ross, L. (1994b) Spiritual aspects of nursing. *Journal of Advanced Nursing*, **19**, 439–447.

Ross, L. (1997) The nurse's role in assessing and responding to patients' spiritual needs. *International Journal of Palliative Nursing*, **3**, 37–42.

Rotter, J. B. (1966) Generalised expectancies for internal versus external control of reinforcement. *Psychological Monographs*, **80**, 1-28.

Rubin, T. I. (1987) When professional help is needed, in *Living Through Personal Crisis*, (ed. A. K. Stearns), Sheldon Press, London.

Sadler, C. (1992) A good death. *Nursing Times*, **88**, 16–17.

Samarel, N. (1995) The dying process, in *Dying: Facing the Facts*, (eds H. Wass and R. A. Neimeyer), Taylor & Francis, Washington, DC, ch. 4, pp. 89–116.

Sarnoff, I. and Corwin, S. M. (1959) Castration anxiety and the fear of death. *Journal of Personality*, **27**, 374–385.

Saunders, J. M. and Valente, S. M. (1994) Nurses' grief. *Cancer Nursing*, **17**, 318–325.

Schmele, J. A. (1995) Perceptions of a dying patient of the quality of care and caring: an interview with Ivan Hanson. *Journal of Nursing Care Quality*, **9**, 31–42.

Schulz, R. and Aderman, D. (1979) Physicians' death anxiety and patient outcomes. *Omega*, **9**, 327–332.

Shanfield, S. B. (1981) The mourning of the health care professional: an important element in education about death and loss. *Death Education*, **4**, 385–395.

Shapiro, C. H. (1988) *Infertility and Pregnancy Loss: A Guide for Helping Professionals*, Jossey-Bass, San Francisco, CA.

Sheard, T. (1984) Dealing with the nurse's grief. *Nursing Forum*, **21**, 43–45.

Shenton, D. (1996) Does aromatherapy provide an holistic approach to palliative care? *International Journal of Palliative Nursing*, **2**, 187–191.

Shields, E. (1994) A daily dose of reflection: developing reflective skills through journal writing. *Professional Nurse*, **9**, 755–758.

Spall, B., Roberts, C. P. and Lewis, S. (1992) A team to tackle the issues that count: problem solving through quality circles. *Professional Nurse*, **7**, 450-452.

Spiegel, Y. (1977) *The Grief Process*, SCM, London.

Stedeford, A. (1981) Couples facing death: II – Unsatisfactory communication. *British Medical Journal*, **283**, 1098–1101.

Stedeford, A. (1984) *Facing Death: Patients, Families and Professionals*, Heinemann, Oxford.

Stewart, A. and Dent, A. (1994) *At a Loss: Bereavement Care When a Baby Dies*, Baillière Tindall, London.

Stroebe, W. and Stroebe M. S. (1987) *Bereavement and Health: The Psychological and Physical Consequences of Partner Loss*, Cambridge University Press, Cambridge.

Sugarman, L. (1986) *Life-Span Development: Concepts, Theories and Interventions*, Routledge, London.

Sutherland, V. J. and Cooper, C. L. (1990) *Understanding Stress: A Psychological Perspective For Health Professionals*, Chapman & Hall, London.

Swanson, T. R. and Swanson, M. J. (1977) Acute uncertainty: the intensive care unit, in *The Experience of Dying*, (ed. E. M. Pattison), Prentice Hall, Englewood Cliffs, NJ.

Taylor, S. E., Lichtman, R. R. and Wood, J. V. (1984) Attributions, beliefs in control, and adjustment to breast cancer. *Journal of Personality and Social Psychology*, **46**, 489–502.

Tedeschi, R. G. and Calhoun, L. G. (1995) *Trauma and Transformation: Growing in the Aftermath of Suffering*, Sage, Thousand Oaks, CA.

Thomas, P. (1995) A study of the effectiveness of staff support groups. *Nursing Times*, **91**, 36–39.

UKCC (1984) Code of Professional Conduct for the Nurse, Midwife and Health Visitor, 2nd edn, UKCC, London.

Vachon, M. L. S. (1987) *Occupational Stress in the Care of the Critically Ill, the Dying and the Bereaved*, Hemisphere, Washington, DC.

Vachon, M. (1988) Battle fatigue in hospice/palliative care, in *A Safer Death: Multidisciplinary Aspects of Terminal Care*, (eds A. Gilmore and S. Gilmore), Plenum Press, London, pp. 149-160.

Ward, B. (1993) *Healing Grief: A Guide to Loss and Recovery*, Vermilion, London.

Ward, B. *et al.* (1993) *Good Grief: Exploring Feelings, Loss and Death with Over Elevens and Adults*, Jessica Kingsley, London.

Warman, J. and Fisher, M. (1990) *Bereavement and Loss – A Skills Companion*, National Extension College, Cambridge.

Warr, P. B. (1987a) *Work, Unemployment and Mental Health*, Oxford University Press, Oxford.

Warr, P. B. (1987b) Workers without a job, in *Psychology At Work*, (ed. P. Warr), Penguin, Harmondsworth, pp. 335-356.

Warwickshire Police (1993) *Breaking Bad News* (video), Warwickshire Police Television Unit.

Weeks, D. (1990) The funeral director and the grieving child, in *The Dying and the Bereaved Teenager*, (ed. J. D. Morgan), Charles Press, Philadelphia, PA, pp. 98-107.

Welch, I. D., Zawistoski, R. F. and Smart, D. W. (1991) *Encountering Death: Structured Activities for Death Awareness*, Accelerated Development Inc., Muncie, IN.

Wells, R. (1988) *Helping Children Cope with Grief: Facing a Death in the Family*, Sheldon Press, London.

Wharton, W. (1994) Wrongful deaths, in *The Sunday Times (The Magazine)*, **16 Oct**.

Whittaker, L. (1995) The cost of caring. Unpublished MA thesis, Keele University.

Wilkinson, S. (1991) Factors which influence how nurses communicate with cancer patients. *Journal of Advanced Nursing*, **16**, 677–688.

Williams, J. (1993) What is a profession? Experience versus expertise, in *Health, Welfare and Practice: Reflecting on Roles and Relationships*, (eds J. Walmsley, J. Reynolds, P. Shakespeare and R. Wolfe), Sage, London.

Wilson, R. (1993) The whirlpool of grief, in *Good Grief: Exploring Feelings, Loss and Death with Over Elevens and Adults* (B. Ward *et al.*), Jessica Kingsley, London.

Worden, J. W. (1991) *Grief Counselling and Grief Therapy: A Handbook for the Mental Health Practitioner*, 2nd edn, Routledge, London.

Wortman, C. B. and Silver, R. C. (1989) The myths of coping with loss. *Journal of Consulting and Clinical Psychology*, **57**, 349–357.

Wright, F. (1988) Lecture given in Macclesfield, Cheshire; see also Wright, F. (1982) The boundaries of life, in *Pastoral Care for Lay People*, SCM, London, ch. 7, pp. 85–96; and Wright, F. (1985) The role of the local church in the healing ministry, in *The Pastoral Nature of Healing*, SCM, London, ch. 4, pp. 49–73.

Wright, B. (1989) Sudden death: nurses' reactions and relatives' opinions. *Bereavement Care*, **8**, 2–4.

Wright, B. (1991) *Sudden Death: Intervention Skills for the Caring Professions*, Churchill Livingstone, Edinburgh.

Wright, B. (1993) *Caring in Crisis: A Handbook of Intervention Skills*, Churchill Livingstone, Edinburgh.

Young, M. and Cullen, L. (1996) *A Good Death: Conversations with East Londoners*, Routledge, London.

Zerwekh, J. Y. (1984) Professional stress and distress, in *Hospice and Palliative Nursing Care*, (eds A. G. Blues and J. Y. Zerwekh), Grune & Stratton, New York, ch. 17, pp. 347–362.

Index